VISION THERAPY IN A PRIMARY-CARE PRACTICE

Jerome Rosner, O.D., F.A.A.O.
Professor
College of Optometry
University of Houston

Joy Rosner, O.D., F.B.C.O.
Assistant Professor
College of Optometry
University of Houston

Professional Press Books
Fairchild Publications
New York

Library of Congress Cataloging-in-Publication Data

Rosner, Jerome.
Vision therapy in a primary-care practice.

Bibliography: p. 143
Includes index.
1. Orthoptics. 2. Eye—Movement disorders—Treatment. I. Rosner, Joy. II. Title. [DNLM: 1. Optometry—methods. 2. Primary Health Care. 3. Vision Disorders—therapy. WW 140 R822v]
RE992.07R67 1988 617.7'62 88-5841
ISBN 0-87873-077-X

Printed in the U.S.A.

Contents

Introduction

This book was written for the primary-care optometrist—the professionally competent practitioner who wants an organized source of information about the use of out-of-office vision therapy in the clinical management of

- Vergence infacility
- Accommodation infacility
- Intermittent strabismus
- Amblyopia
- Constant strabismus
- Perceptual skills dysfunction

The information presented here is meant to be practical rather than scientific. It describes a systematic, easy-to-apply method that the optometrist can use to incorporate vision therapy into a busy primary-care practice without making significant investments in office space, personnel, equipment, or time.

The format of the book is highly structured. To some, in fact, it may seem too mechanical, too much like a cookbook. We take the opposite view. Because its format is so structured, the book highlights clearly the principles that are central to the management of out-of-office vision therapy programs in a primary-care optometric practice. Vision therapy is not an art. It is based on an organized set of definable principles and empirical data, as are refraction and contact lens fitting. (True, there is the art of interacting with patients, but that applies to all clinical aspects of the profession, not just to vision therapy.) Hence, the benefits of the format far outweigh any drawbacks.

Chapter 1, "Guidelines for Implementing a Vision Therapy Program," explicates the concepts that are fundamental to the organization of this book and describes how they are applied. The reader is shown an orderly process for making treatment decisions and, when vision therapy is prescribed, how to design a treatment regimen as a sequence of hierarchically interrelated behavioral goals that will serve as both tests and treatment objectives. This makes it possible for the therapy program to be organized as a set of repetitive (in-office) skills testing and (out-of-office) skills training episodes that methodically lead the patient to a final goal, step by step.

Chapters 2 through 7 center on the six clinical conditions listed above. All six chapters have a similar structure. Each is divided into three major sections: identification, treatment and representative case reports. These major sections, in turn, follow the same organization in each of the chapters.

Chapter 8 is devoted to management. It addresses such topics as training of office personnel, instruments, materials, fees, and effective use of office space. (All the instruments are inexpensive, readily obtainable from United States sources, and easy to transport between the optometrist's office and the patient's home.)

The Bibliography is organized according to topic and identifies sources of additional pertinent information. The reading list is not exhaustive, but it will serve the interested reader effectively.

A separate volume—the Procedures Manual—contains all the therapy procedures cited in this book and a copy of a daily log on which the patient records his progress.* The procedures are written in an unambiguous, directive style. They tell the patient what to do, how to do it, and what to pay attention to as he is doing it. Each procedure has been designed so that it and the daily log, once photocopied, may be modified when called for to meet a patient's unique needs, and dispensed for home use with a minimum of explanation. Also in this manual are a copy of the Test of Visual Analysis Skills (TVAS) and certain other related materials. These, too, may be reproduced for office use.

ORGANIZATION OF CHAPTERS 2, 3, 4, 5, 6, and 7

Each of these clinical-condition chapters is organized as follows:

IDENTIFICATION

How to identify those patients who manifest the condition under discussion and how to decide who among them are good candidates for vision therapy. This comprises three sections.

Signs and symptoms of the condition
Prevalence of the condition
Screening tests

---

* For the purpose of clear communication, certain conventions are followed throughout this book: The patient is referred to as *he;* the optometrist is referred to as *he or she;* and when discussion deals with patient decisions or responsibilities, it is assumed that the patient will take on these obligations when appropriate.

TREATMENT

What to recommend and how to implement that recommendation within the practical constraints of a typical primary-care practice. This, too, is organized in three sections.

Factors the Optometrist Should Consider

Prognosis for Remediation Through Vision Therapy. The effectiveness of vision therapy depends upon the nature of the condition being treated and certain patient attributes. In regard to the latter, the optometrist is well advised to remember and to inform the patient that vision therapy is not treatment in the sense of a medical model. The cause of the patient's problem will probably not be identified and then eliminated. Nor is vision therapy analogous to a physical fitness program, in which muscles are made stronger. Vision therapy is an *educational* process; the patient must learn something rather than be cured of a disease.

Effective vision therapy provides circumstances that enable the patient to learn a new (desirable) behavior that replaces an existing (undesirable) behavior. That goal can be achieved only if the patient has the physiological, intellectual, and motivational traits needed to learn how to perform a specified behavior under controlled, supportive conditions, with feedback informing him when he is performing correctly; match what he feels (intrinsic cues) with that feedback (extrinsic cues); and finally, perform the newly learned behavior automatically, without conscious effort, even when the (extrinsic) feedback is eliminated—in short, to replace a bad habit with a good habit.

The process depends upon the inductive learning that occurs as the patient becomes adept at performing new behaviors. Some patients are not able to benefit from such self-instruction, perhaps because of their immaturity, perhaps because of an unwillingness to devote sufficient time to practicing what they are learning, or perhaps because of other limitations. The treatment recommendations should reflect this.*

Alternative treatment options. Vision therapy is not the treatment of choice in all cases. Some patients should be managed differently. Each of the chapters dealing with a specific clinical problem contains a section devoted to alternative treatment options and their relative advantages and disadvantages. These options are

Reassurance Informing the patient that, for him, benign neglect—leaving well enough alone—is the best treatment, at least in the short term; that there is no risk inherent in such an approach—the condition will not worsen; and that a more active treatment may be called for in the future, as determined at subsequent visits.

Referral Suggesting consultation with someone able to provide additional information relevant to the patient's condition. In some cases, the referral should be made to an optometrist who specializes in vision therapy; in others, to a surgeon, a psychologist, or other professional.

Compensation Some patients lack the time, motivation, cognitive ability, or physiological capacity needed to benefit from vision therapy. They will not be

---

* There is no upper-age limit so long as the patient has the traits mentioned above.

helped by vision therapy although others with similar problems have been successfully treated that way. These individuals should be provided with a compensatory device or some other type of accommodation that enables them to function adequately—or as close to it as possible—despite the problem.

Factors the Patient Should Consider

Probable outcome of treatment Potential benefits and risks from the patient's point of view

Obligations The time and effort that the treatment will require

Consequences (short-term and long-term) if the recommendation for vision therapy is not accepted

Number and frequency of office visits

Implementation of Vision Therapy

Steps to be taken once the patient decides to accept a recommendation for vision therapy.

CASE REPORTS

Examples of how the condition under discussion was treated—presenting symptoms, salient clinical data, decisions, treatments prescribed, and outcomes.

END OF FIRST VISIT

All the events described above, under Identification and Treatment, usually take place during the patient's first visit. If vision therapy is prescribed and if the patient accepts the recommendation, he should be scheduled for a second visit. This second visit will probably be managed by the office assistant, either exclusively or almost so. Indeed, once the first visit has been completed, about 80 to 90 percent of the vision therapy patient's office time should be assigned to the office assistant, with the optometrist's involvement being limited to consulting, responding to problems that might arise, reassuring, and so on. Chapter 1 describes the format of the second and subsequent visits.

CHAPTER 1

Guidelines for Implementing a Vision Therapy Program

THE SECOND VISIT

Once the patient has accepted a recommendation for vision therapy, certain preparatory steps should be taken. These typically occur at the second visit and are carried out by the office assistant.

1. Administer placement tests to document what skills the patient already has (in the context of what he is to learn) and what yet remains to be achieved.

RATIONALE FOR PLACEMENT TESTING PROTOCOL

Fundamental to the placement-test process is the specification of the ultimate and subordinate goals of the therapy program. This is accomplished as follows:

In each of the chapters that focus on a specific clinical condition (chapters 2 and 7), the ultimate goal of the therapy program is defined in behavioral terms—what the patient will be able to do upon completion of the therapy if the program is successful.

The purpose of stating the ultimate goal in behavioral terms is that, as already noted, vision therapy is an educational, not a curative, process. If the optometrist is to succeed in the role of teacher, he or she should be able to state just what it is that the patient is to learn and how he will be able to demonstrate (to the optometrist and to himself) that he has learned it.

The implication of the ultimate goal is that achieving it promises the elimination (or marked reduction) of the signs and symptoms that originally precipitated the treatment effort. To ensure this, the ultimate goals of the different therapy programs depicted in this book are significantly more demanding than the screening test criteria used to identify the condition. This is done to overtrain the patient—to make sure that the skills he is working on are overlearned to the point where they are performed automatically, virtually without conscious effort.

In each of these chapters, the goals that subserve the ultimate goal of the therapy program are also defined in behavioral terms and then organized according to their levels of relative difficulty and interdependence. In many instances, this requires some arbitrary determinations. See, for example, the subordinate goals of the vergence infacility program (chapter 2, pp. 10–11). Identifying subordinate goals serves an important purpose. Because they are stated in behavioral terms and organized according to relative difficulty, they can be used both to assess the patient's entering abilities and as milestones for documenting subsequent progress.

TO ADMINISTER PLACEMENT TESTS

Start with the level I goals of the program. Regardless of which condition is being treated or which therapy program is being implemented, this represents the least demanding level in the sequence. If the patient meets the criteria of level I goals, test him on the goals of level II, and so on upward until failure is demonstrated.

The patient is placed in the level in which he failed to meet the requirements of the goal. For example, if the patient passes (meets criteria defined by the stated goals of) levels I and II, then fails level III goals, he is placed in level III. That becomes the starting point of his therapy program. He is assigned activities that will help him achieve the goals of level III.

2. *During placement testing, in preparation for selecting an appropriate skills training procedure, pay special attention to differences in performance the patient may display as a function of such factors as:*

FIXATION DISTANCE

Some patients have much more difficulty performing a visual behavior at distance than at near (e.g., vergence facility, accommodation facility, single simultaneous binocular vision); with others, the reverse may be true. If the patient shows a marked preference, therapy should begin at the fixation distance that causes him the least difficulty, with the more demanding condition being introduced as progress allows. If no major difference is observed, then this factor may be ignored when procedures are selected.

DIRECTION OF VERGENCE OR ACCOMMODATION ADAPTATION

Some patients have much more difficulty exercising positive relative convergence facility (meeting base-out demands) than they do exercising negative relative convergence facility (meeting base-in demands); others, vice versa. Similarly, some patients have more difficulty activating accommodation (i.e., adapting to minus lenses); others, inhibiting accommodation (i.e., adapting to plus lenses). If the patient shows a marked preference, therapy should begin with the type of demand that presents the least difficulties. If no major difference is observed, then this factor may be ignored when therapy procedures are selected.

COMPENSATORY SPHERES OR PRISMS

Some patients need compensatory lenses (spheres or prisms) in order to get started in a vision therapy procedure. This is particularly true of patients with constant strabismus, but also applies to those with less complex binocular problems. For example, patients with high esophoria or intermittent esotropia will frequently get off to a better start if they are given extra plus spheres in bifocal form for near fixation. In some cases, the effect may be further enhanced by providing some base-out prisms as well. Similarly, patients manifesting significant exophoria or intermittent exotropia often have less difficulty getting started in a procedure if they are supplied with minus lenses or base-in prisms. If this type of support appears to be called for, it should be supplied, then withdrawn as the patient makes progress and demonstrates that the support is no longer needed.*

3. *Select the procedure(s) that will teach the patient the skills he needs to learn next to reduce the separation between his present status and what is called for by the ultimate goal of his therapy program.* Do this on the basis of the placement testing, but where relevant, keep in mind, also, the factors mentioned above: relative effects of fixation distance, direction of adaptation, and the relative usefulness of compensatory spheres or prisms. Each of chapters 2 through 7 contains a table that identifies appropriate procedures. The procedures themselves are located in numerical order in the Procedures Manual.

RATIONALE FOR DESIGN OF PROCEDURES

All the procedures cited in this book conform to a set of instructional principles. When used correctly, the procedures are

Instructive, teach the patient a behavior he currently cannot perform, is now ready to learn (in respect to prerequisite skills), and needs to learn in order to make progress toward the ultimate goal of the treatment program.

Modifiable in terms of relative difficulty: It is possible to make an activity easier by providing additional support if the patient requires and reversing the situation as the patient gains competence.

Quantifiable, capable of being expressed in fairly specific terms.

Self-instructional: The patient is able to monitor his own performance rather than having to depend on someone else for that information—initially through overt feedback (what he sees) that is matched to intrinsic cues (what he feels), later through intrinsic cues alone.

Effective, capable, in time, of replacing an undesirable habitual behavior with a desirable habitual behavior.

4. *Locate the procedure and photocopy it.*

---

* These factors pertain to patients with binocular dysfunction; they may not be relevant in cases of perceptual skills dysfunction (see chapter 7).

5. *Amend the procedure to make it more or less difficult, in accord with the patient's needs and the treatment goals.* Each printed procedure has a section of special instructions for this purpose. Say, for example, that the patient manifests esophoria, vergence infacility, and moderate hyperopia (Rx: (OU) +1.25 D spheres). He is about to begin therapy to improve vergence facility, with special emphasis on building up his ability to exercise negative relative convergence at nearpoint (meet base-in demands). At the onset, it will be easier for the patient to work through some of the activities if he wears his glasses—and perhaps even easier if he is supplied with some extra plus spheres (e.g., +1.00 D) to use in addition to his own glasses as he begins a procedure (see case report of patient 2.2, visit 3; p. 17). In time, of course, the extra plus spheres will be eliminated—perhaps gradually, perhaps abruptly, depending upon the kind of support he needs in order to progress. In fact, it may even be that later on the patient will be assigned the same procedure, but this time while wearing minus spheres (as training glasses) to make the activities even more demanding. In essence, then, one amends a procedure to make it easier or more difficult by introducing spheres or prisms. Tailoring the procedure in this way enables it to be employed more effectively over a wider range of applications.

6. *Instruct the patient in the implementation of the procedure and the keeping of the daily log.* Ordinarily, this involves taking the patient through the mechanics of the activity step-by-step, making sure that he will be able to accomplish the beginning activities without confusion or undue difficulty after he leaves the office. To ensure this, the patient should *do* the prescribed activity in the presence of the office assistant—assemble the apparatus (if one is called for) and carry out the beginning steps of the procedure, not just talk about it.

7. *Enter any relevant observations into the patient's record: for example, "diplopia experienced at 2 PD base out."*

8. *Stress to the patient the importance of following the instructions, not only in respect to what he is to do but also how often and for how long he is to do it.*

9. *Emphasize to the patient the importance of learning through doing, thinking about what he is doing and how it feels and relating this to what he sees.*

10. *Schedule the follow-up visit.* The frequency of visits may vary with the different clinical conditions and is therefore discussed separately in each of the chapters.

11. *Assure the patient that he is to telephone if questions or problems arise before his next visit.*

FOLLOW-UP VISITS

At each subsequent follow-up visit, the office assistant should

1. Obtain information from the patient (and his daily log) regarding what has occurred since the last visit. For example: Did he comply with the prescribed schedule? Where any problems encountered; if so, were they solved and how? How much progress was made in terms of the printed instructions? Were any

positive or negative effects noted (e.g., discomfort or increased comfort, diplopia or reduction of diplopia, increased or decreased difficulty as the procedure was practiced).

2. Re-administer the placement tests, beginning with the test for the level in which the patient was placed at the previous visit. For example, say the patient was placed in level I at the last visit: this means that he could not accomplish the goal(s) of that level. At the subsequent visit, re-test for that level. If it has been accomplished, test the next higher level in the sequence, and so on. If it has not been accomplished, follow the guidelines given below.

3. Select and photocopy a new procedure that is appropriate for the level defined by the placement re-testing just completed. (This presumes that the patient has progressed beyond the level of the previous visit. If he has not, follow the guidelines suggested below.)

4. Amend the procedure (in the special-instructions section of the printed handout) to make it more or less demanding, as described above, and go through it with the patient.

5. Schedule subsequent follow-up visits in accord with the typical regimen suggested in the chapter that pertains to the condition under therapy.

IF THE PATIENT DOES NOT MAKE EXPECTED PROGRESS

If the patient does not make sufficient progress, if he does not achieve the goal(s) of the level in which he was placed, ascertain whether this is because of a lack of adherence to the daily schedule or, rather, some confusion about what he was to do. If it is the latter, have him demonstrate what he has been doing. If, indeed, the instructions were followed correctly, the optometrist or office assistant should do one or both of the following:

1. Reassure the patient that all that is needed is more time or effort at this level (this often occurs with constant strabismics, who may remain in level I for a long time).
2. Select and prescribe a different procedure that might be more motivating.

IF THE PATIENT DOES NOT COMPLY

If it is established that the patient did not adhere to the daily schedule, one of two options should be considered. In either case, the optometrist, not the office assistant, should communicate with the patient at this point.

1. Offer a second chance, but only if convinced that the patient is likely to alter his behavior this time.
2. Discontinue the treatment program and suggest one of the alternative treatment options described above (i.e., reassurance, referral, or a compensatory device). This should not be done under the guise of punishment. Rather, it should be presented to the patient as recognition of the fact that conditions may not be correct for such an undertaking at this time.

CHAPTER 2

Vergence Infacility

Efficient visual functioning depends on more than 20/20 acuity and binocular alignment. If the patient is capable of single simultaneous binocular vision, some attention should be given to his ability to maintain that bifoveal alignment under dynamic, stressful conditions. Traditionally, the optometrist comes close to assessing this with tests of positive and negative relative convergence (i.e., base-in and base-out fusional reserves) at distance and near. These are well-established, useful tests, but they fail to take *facility* into account, the patient's ability to adapt quickly and easily to abrupt changes in vergence demands while holding accommodation constant. The term *vergence infacility* refers to those patients who, although binocular, lack this capacity.

IDENTIFICATION

Signs and Symptoms

These assume that the patient has been wearing whatever lenses he needs to compensate fully for any existing ametropia. Not all of the following are necessarily displayed or experienced by all patients.

1. Discomfort (fatigue, headaches, eyestrain, etc.) during or following prolonged visual activity
2. Avoidance of close work
3. Significant (horizontal or vertical) heterophoria at one or more fixation distances, sometimes not apparent until the patient is fatigued or unless the

phoria is measured after a relatively long period of disassociation by either prism or occluder

4. Reduced fusional vergence ranges in one or more directions

5. Slow adaptation to abrupt changes in vergence demands, especially when accommodation is held constant

6. Unstable binocularity, with or without occasional diplopia

Prevalence

Exceptionally high in all age groups.

Screening Tests

To be conducted with patient wearing whatever lenses needed to compensate fully for existing ametropia.

Vergence Facility at Distance

1. Patient fixates on a vertical row of small but legible letters (about 20/20 to 20/30) located 6 m away. Examiner makes certain that the patient sees the letters singly and clearly. A vertical row of letters is best because if diplopia is provoked, it will be more apparent to the patient under these conditions than with a horizontal row of letters.

2. Hold a 6 diopter (D) prism, base-in, before patient's right or left eye and ask, *"How many rows of letters do you see now?"* If patient reports seeing two, say, *"Try to get them together and tell me as soon as they merge into a single row and become clear."* Watch the patient's eyes to confirm objectively what he is reporting. The fusional vergence movements should be very apparent.

3. If, and as soon as, fusion and clarity are obtained, remove the prism, again asking the patient to report when the row of letters is single and clear.

4. As soon as patient reports fusion and clarity without prism, re-introduce the base-in prism, repeating step 2. As before, watch the patient's eyes to confirm his reports. Continue in this manner until the patient has successfully accomplished three cycles or until 30 seconds have elapsed, whichever occurs first. A cycle consists of, first, fusion and clarity without prism, then fusion and clarity with prism, then again without prism. Consider three cycles within 30 seconds to be satisfactory (passing) performance (see criteria below).

5. If the patient satisfies criterion (i.e., three cycles accomplished within 30 seconds), go to step 7.

6. If the patient does not satisfy criterion, reduce prism power in 2 D increments and repeat procedure until he is able to execute three cycles within 30 seconds. Then, to rule out the possibility that the patient may simply have been a bit slow in understanding what he was to do, continue testing as you increase prism power in 2 D increments until threshold (or the capacity to deal successfully with a 6 D base-in prism) is reached. Record the power of that prism. For example, if initially the patient could not manage the 6 D nor the 4 D base-in prism but

could deal successfully with the 2 D prism, re-test with the 4 D prism. If he passes, go up to 6 prism diopters (PD) and if he now displays the ability to accomplish three cycles with that power within 30 seconds, record a passing performance with the 6 D prism. Then go to step 7.

7. Repeat the process with base-out prisms, starting with 12 PD.

Vergence Facility at Near

Repeat the far-point procedures described above, this time using a vertical row of small letters held at 40 cm. Measure base-in facility first, starting with 12 PD; then base-out, starting with 14 PD.

Performance Criteria. These have been established arbitrarily but appear to be clinically valid. In effect, they are comparable to the recovery measures of positive and negative relative convergence when tested in the standard way (i.e., with Risley prisms in a phoropter).

Consider the following to be indicative of satisfactory vergence facility:

AT FAR	Base in: Plano to 6 PD*
	Base out: Plano to 12 PD*
AT NEAR	Base in: Plano to 12 PD*
	Base out: Plano to 14 PD*

Obviously, if the optometrist believes that a patient does not manifest vergence infacility despite failure on the screening test, or vice versa—if the optometrist believes that the patient does manifest vergence infacility despite having passed the screening test—then, as always, professional judgment takes precedence. In general, however, the criteria stated above will discriminate accurately.

TREATMENT

Factors the Optometrist Should Consider

Prognosis for Remediation Through Vision Therapy. Very favorable, especially if the patient displays precise bifoveal alignment (i.e., better than 100 sec of arc stereoacuity at far, better than 60 sec at near). Prognosis is relatively less favorable if stereoacuity is poor, but therapy is probably still worthwhile (see chapters 4 and 6).

Alternative Treatment Options

Reassurance Benign neglect of vergence infacility is not recommended. The condition does not often deteriorate into a markedly worse condition (e.g., intermittent or constant strabismus), but it could. Even if it does not worsen, it is not likely to disappear; the patient's symptoms will remain.

---

* Three cycles within 30 seconds

Referral There is rarely any need for consultation in such cases once the possibility of pathology and structural anomaly has been ruled out.

Compensation If the patient does not display the intellectual, physiological, or motivational traits needed to profit from vision therapy, consider prescribing compensatory lenses (prisms or spheres) to reduce some of the stress the patient faces when engaging in demanding visual activities (base-in prism when positive relative convergence facility is deficient; base-out prism—or some additional plus spheres for near, in the form of bifocals—when negative relative convergence facility is deficient; base down for hyperphoria, etc.). This will not eliminate the problem, but it will enable the patient to engage in visual activities more comfortably despite the functional deficit. How much prism or spherical power? That will vary with the case, but as a rule of thumb, use enough power to put into balance the relationship between the patient's phorias and his—base-in and base-out, base-up and base-down—fusional reserves.

Factors the Patient Should Consider

Probable Outcome of Treatment. An improved capacity to engage comfortably in sustained visual activities.

Consequences If Recommendations Are Not Followed. A lack of compliance will probably result in the continuation of present symptoms or the need for compensatory treatment. It is not likely to result in a significantly worsened visual status.

Patient's Obligations. The patient will probably be required to devote about 15 to 30 minutes to prescribed remedial activities daily for approximately four to eight weeks. This will be followed by four months or so of maintenance activities that require about 2 to 5 minutes per day.

Number and Frequency of Office Visits. Patient should anticipate between four and nine visits, depending on the level where therapy begins and the rate at which he progresses. More specifically, if the patient begins therapy in level I (see below), successful treatment of vergence infacility, on average, probably requires from six to nine office visits. If he places in level II, treatment usually requires about two fewer office visits. If the patient places in level III or higher, treatment is not likely to require more than three to five office visits.

Implementation of Vision Therapy

Steps to be taken once the patient elects to accept the recommendation for vision therapy:

1. Schedule Patient for a Second Visit. At that visit, the office assistant will carry out the sequence of procedures described in chapter 1 (pp. 1–4), commencing with placement testing.

TABLE 2.1 Vergence Facility Treatment Goals

	Prism power (PD)				
	Far		Near		
Level	**Base in**	**Base out**	**Base in**	**Base out**	**Cycle**[a]
IV	6	12	12	14	Base in to base out to base in
III	4	6	8	8	Base in to base out to base in
II	2	4	4	6	Base in to base out to base in
I	3	3	6	6	Plano to prism to plano
	Patient experiences physiological diplopia immediately upon being presented with appropriate conditions.				

[a] Rate = 60 cycles with 5 minutes

2. Placement Testing. Levels and goals, organized in descending order of difficulty (see also Table 2.1).

LEVEL IV

This is the final goal: Patient is able to execute fusional vergence jumps as follows:

AT FAR From 6 PD base in *to* 12 PD base out, and vice versa,* *and*
AT NEAR From 12 PD base in *to* 14 PD base out, and vice versa*

LEVEL III

Patient is able to execute fusional vergence jumps as follows:

AT FAR From 4 PD base in *to* 6 PD base out, and vice versa,* *and*
AT NEAR From 8 PD base in *to* 8 PD base out, and vice versa*

Test at far, then at near.

LEVEL II

AT FAR From 2 PD base in *to* 4 PD base out, and vice versa,* *and*
AT NEAR From 4 PD base in *to* 6 PD base out, and vice versa*

Test at far, then at near.

* Sixty cycles within 5 minutes. For one cycle, start with fusion and clarity through base-in prism (unmounted, hand-held, or mounted in flippers), then fusion and clarity through base-out prism, then again through base-in.

LEVEL I

There are two goals for this level:

a. Patient is able to execute fusional vergence jumps as follows:

AT FAR	From 3 PD base in *to* plano, and vice versa,* *and*
	From 3 PD base out *to* plano, and vice versa,* *and*
AT NEAR	From 6 PD base in *to* plano, and vice versa*
	From 6 PD base out *to* plano, and vice versa*

b. Patient experiences and reports physiological diplopia immediately upon being presented with appropriate stimuli and conditions (e.g., a row of letters at 6 m and a penlight at 40 cm).

3. Patient's Performance. During placement testing, pay special attention to differences in performance the patient may display as a function of

Fixation distance As pointed out in chapter 1, if the patient has significantly more difficulty at one fixation distance than at another (i.e., far versus near), he should commence therapy with the least demanding condition, the other being introduced as progress allows. If no major difference is observed, then start where it is most convenient.

Direction of the vergence adaptation Some patients have much more difficulty meeting the demands of base-out prism than they do base-in prism; others, vice versa. If the patient shows a marked preference, therapy should begin with the type of vergence demand that presents the least difficulties. If no major difference is observed, then start where it is most convenient.

4. Select Procedure. Select appropriate procedure(s) from Table 2.2., keeping in mind the two factors mentioned above (i.e., relative difficulty of near versus far fixation distance and direction of vergence adaptation). Locate the procedure and photocopy it.

5. Amend the Procedure. Amend the procedure in the special-instructions section of the printed handout to make it more or less demanding, in accord with the patient's needs and the treatment goals. For example, a patient with a moderate degree of hyperopia will have relatively less difficulty with far-point base-out demand activities if he does not wear his glasses; hence, such an activity may be made a bit easier for him if the special-instructions section of the procedure advises that he start off without his glasses, then repeat the activities while he wears his glasses. Conversely, a myope is likely to have relatively less difficulty with near-point base-out demand activities if he wears his glasses, and more difficulty if he does not wear them.

---

* Sixty cycles within 5 minutes. For one cycle, start with fusion and clarity without prism then fusion and clarity through base-in prism (loose, hand-held, or mounted in flippers); then again fusion and clarity when prism is removed. Repeat with base-out prism.

TABLE 2.2 Vergence Facility Procedures

Procedure	Apparatus	This procedure is appropriate if the patient is to start therapy at/with: Far	Near	Base in	Base out	Prerequisites[a]
1	Aperture rule; target cards; aperture slides		X	X	X	A
2	Aperture rule; target cards		X	X	X	A, E
3-I	Eccentric rectangle targets		X	X	X	A, E
3-II	Eccentric rectangle targets	X		X	X	B, E
3-III	Eccentric rectangle targets	X	X	X	X	A, B, E
4	Variable-mirror stereoscope; stereo targets		X	X	X	A, E
5	Brewster stereoscope; Adult Base-Out Comfort Series	X			X	B
6	Brewster stereoscope; Keystone Children's Base-Out Stories	X			X	B
7	Brewster stereoscope; Keystone Children's Base-In Stories	X		X		B
8	Minivectograms; polarizers		X	X	X	A, E
9	Minitranaglyphs; red-green filters		X	X	X	A, E
10	Vectotrainer; quoit vectograms; polarizers		X	X	X	A, E
11	Any nonvariable-disparity tranaglyph; red-green filters		X	X	X	A, E
12	Brewster stereoscope; Bernell Base-Out Story Book Cards	X			X	B
13	Brewster stereoscope; Bernell Base-In Story Book Cards	X		X		B
14	Any variable-disparity vectograms; polarizers		X	X	X	A, E
15	Any variable-disparity tranaglyphs; red-green filters		X	X	X	A, E
16	Red-green stereo trainer; red-green filters; horizontal prisms	X	X	X	X	A, B
17	Red-green stereo trainer; red-green filters; vertical prisms	X	X			A, B
18	Vertical minivectograms; polarizers		X			A

TABLE 2.2 (Continued)

Proce-dure	Apparatus	This procedure is appropriate if the patient is to start therapy at/with Far	Near	Base in	Base out	Prerequi-sites[a]
19	Brock string; targets	X	X			C, D
20	Two fixation targets; red filter	X	X			C, D
21	Phy-Dip Stick		X			C

[a] Prerequisites: A = third-degree fusion (i.e., stereopsis) at near; B = third-degree fusion at far; C = second-degree fusion at near; D = second-degree fusion at far; E = well-established awareness of physiological diplopia.

6. Postplacement Testing. Continue with the postplacement testing sequence as described in chapter 1 (pp. 1–4).

Very little mention has been made in this chapter regarding the treatment of patients with vertical heterophoria and inadequate adaptive (fusional) ranges. The same treatment principles apply for them; the same four treatment options should be considered. If vision therapy is the treatment of choice, see Table 2.2 and procedures manual for suggested procedures.

CASE REPORTS

Patient 2.1—Exophoria with Vergence Infacility

VISIT 1

Patient is a 12-year-old, sixth grader.

Chief Complaints Discomfort at extended near work; early onset of fatigue; diplopia (rarely) when extremely tired.

Salient Clinical Data *Health status:* No evidence of pathology

Visual acuity: 20/20 each eye at distance and near

Refractive status: Emmetropia

Binocular status

AT FAR 4 PD exophoria
Stereoacuity: 1 min of arc
Vergence Facility: Can recover fusion through 6 PD base in, but only 4 PD base out.

AT NEAR 12 PD exophoria
Stereoacuity: 40 sec of arc
Near-point convergence: 11 in
Vergence facility: Can recover fusion through 12 PD base in, but only 6 PD base out

All else within normal limits.

Conclusion Patient's symptoms appear to derive from vergence infacility.

Prescription Either compensatory (base-in) prism spectacles or vision therapy. The latter is recommended. Patient accepts recommendation and is scheduled for second visit.

VISIT 2 (ONE WEEK LATER)

Placement Testing Placement testing always starts with level I goals. Patient shows mastery of level I goals but fails level II. He has no difficulty regaining fusion through the low-power prisms (of level II goal) but is unable to execute 60 cycles within 5 minutes at far or at near. (He was able to complete about 20 cycles, but then fatigue set in and performance deteriorated.) Therefore, placement is in level II; therapy begins at this level.

Procedure 1 is selected, photocopied, and dispensed as is (i.e., nothing added to the special-instructions section) along with a daily log form and an aperture rule. Because the patient did not have more or less difficulty at far fixation than at near, this factor did not influence the decision regarding procedure; however, because the patient encountered more difficulty meeting base-out prism demands (as compared with base-in) but could already maintain fusion through moderate amounts of base-out prism, the decision was made to start off with a procedure that called for the exercising of positive relative convergence. Hence, any of the procedures in Table 2.2 that are designated as being appropriate for improving base-out ranges could have been prescribed. Procedure 1 was selected simply as a matter of convenience.

VISIT 3 (TWO WEEKS LATER)

Patient reports, and daily log shows, satisfactory completion of procedure 1, but symptoms persist. In fact, they may be worse. His eyes *"feel tired, even hurt sometimes,"* especially just after he has completed a therapy session.

Re-administration of placement tests indicates that patient is able to meet the goals of level II, but not level III. Patient is assured that he has made progress and that his symptoms are not unusual.

Procedure 2 is selected (from Table 2.2), photocopied, and dispensed to the patient unamended along with a new daily log form and the aperture rule, but this time without the aperture slides. (Again, any of the procedures listed in the table could have been used. Procedure 2 was selected because it follows nicely after procedure 1; very little additional patient orientation is needed.)

VISIT 4 (TWO WEEKS LATER)

Patient reports almost satisfactory completion of procedure 2; that is, he can accomplish the jumps called for by the instructions but has difficulty maintaining the rate. Symptoms have diminished; patient is able to read for longer periods without experiencing discomfort.

Re-administration of placement tests corroborates patient's report. He cannot achieve the goals of level III, not because of an inability to execute the vergence jumps, but, rather, because of an inability to maintain required rate of 60 cycles within 5 minutes.

A new procedure (3-I) is dispensed to patient along with a pair of near-point targets (eccentric rectangles) and, of course, a new daily log.

It would have been acceptable to continue the patient with the procedure that was dispensed at the previous visit, but a new procedure was introduced because all his treatment, to date, had been carried out at near point. This new procedure leads easily to an effective far-point procedure (3-II). In addition, vergence infacility cases are usually completed with procedure 3-III because

1. The equipment is expendable.
2. A special setting is not required: the patient can engage in the activity whenever and wherever he has a few spare minutes.
3. The activity is versatile: it may be carried out at any fixation distance—near, far, or in between.
4. The activity may be used to enhance base-in or base-out prism facility with equal effectiveness.
5. The activity is carried out in real space; therefore its effects are readily transferred into the patient's everyday environments and activities.

VISIT 5 (TEN DAYS LATER)

Patient reports satisfactory completion of procedure 3-I. Symptoms, for the most part, have disappeared, manifesting only when patient is very fatigued.

Re-administration of placement tests corroborates patient's report. He is able to demonstrate the goal of Level III; however, he has not yet acquired the abilities called for by the level IV goal.

A new procedure (3-II) is dispensed to patient.

VISIT 6 (TWO WEEKS LATER)

Patient reports satisfactory completion of procedure 3-II. Symptoms have disappeared.

Re-administration of placement tests corroborates patient's report. He is able to demonstrate the goal of level IV without difficulty. All that remains is for the patient to continue to practice this final behavior daily for the next three to four months to the point where he can perform the behaviors automatically, virtually without conscious effort. Patient is advised accordingly and given unamended procedure 3-III; in effect, this procedure merges the two previous ones (3-I and 3-II) into a single, highly effective activity.

VISIT 7 (THREE MONTHS LATER)

Patient has complied with instructions; he has practiced the final procedure (3-III) daily since his last visit. Patient symptom-free.

Re-administration of placement tests indicates that patient has acquired excellent vergence facility at both distance and near. Patient is advised to continue to practice final activity about once a week until he returns for his next routine annual examination. Case successfully completed.

Patient 2.2—Esophoria with Vergence Infacility

VISIT 1

Patient is a 22-year-old college student.

Chief Complaints

Fatigue at close work; occasional diplopia at near, especially when he does not wear his glasses (habitual lens Rx: (OU) +1.00 D spheres). Patient has had these glasses for five years but never wore them very much. Lately, he has noticed that they do help with close work and has been wearing them more often.

Salient Clinical Data

Health status: No evidence of pathology
Visual acuity: 20/20 each eye at distance and near (with and without glasses)
Refractive status: (OU) +1.25 D spheres
Binocular status

AT FAR — 2 PD esophoria without glasses; orthophoria with glasses
Stereoacuity: 1 min of arc (with and without glasses)
Vergence facility: Fails screening test; cannot regain fusion through more than 3 PD base in; passes base-out component
Accommodation facility: Fails, diplopia through −1.50 D spheres

AT NEAR — 8 PD esophoria without glasses; orthophoria with glasses
Stereoacuity: 40 sec of arc with or without glasses
Vergence facility: Fails, cannot regain fusion through more than 4 PD base in; passes base-out component
Accommodation facility: Fails, cannot clear through powers in excess of −1.00 D spheres (OU)

All else within normal limits.

Conclusion

Patient's symptoms are attributable to high esophoria in combination with a high AC/A ratio and vergence infacility.

Prescription

Patient is advised that his symptoms and problem can be treated in one of two ways: (1) by wearing glasses that provide additional plus power for near work, this in the form of bifocal lenses, or (2) by engaging in vision therapy, which would not free him from the need for glasses, especially for close work, but probably would eliminate the need for the bifocal lenses. Patient not happy about the idea of bifocals and chooses to try vision therapy. Patient is scheduled for second visit.

VISIT 2 (THREE DAYS LATER)

Placement Testing

Decision was made to ignore accommodation infacility and to concentrate on vergence infacility, at least at the onset, because as patient acquires more acceptable fusional vergence ranges, accommodation facility should also improve. Approaching the problem from the opposite end, that is, by addressing the accommodation infacility first, would probably have been just as reasonable.

Patient fails level I goals. He cannot meet the base-in prism requirements of that level, even when wearing his glasses, nor is he able to appreciate physiological diplopia. Hence, placement is in level I; therapy begins at this level.

Procedures 19 (physiological diplopia) and 13 are selected, photocopied, and dispensed to the patient along with a Brewster stereoscope and the Base-In Story Book Cards.

Procedure 13 was chosen because (1) the patient had significantly less difficulty at far than at near fixation; and (2) although the patient's main limitation was with base-in prism, he had no difficulty with base-out prism, he was able to meet moderate base-in demands. Procedures 7 or 16 would also have satisfied his condition. An entry was made into the special-instructions section of the procedure 13 handout advising the patient to first work through all the activities while wearing his glasses, then to go through them again without glasses.

VISIT 3 (TWO WEEKS LATER)

Patient's daily log shows satisfactory completion of the two procedures, both while wearing and while not wearing his glasses. Symptoms persist.

Re-administration of placement tests indicates that patient now can meet the goals of level I (with or without his glasses), but not level II. Patient is assured that progress is being made.

Procedure 8 is selected (from Table 2.2), photocopied, and dispensed to the patient along with the minivectograms.

This procedure focuses on near-point facility. Not surprisingly, patient displayed some difficulty with this procedure when it was dispensed, even when he wore his glasses. For this reason, the procedure was amended in the special-instructions section to incorporate the use of loaned +2.00 D sphere (OU) training glasses that he was to wear in lieu of his own glasses until he started to make headway. Then, he was to switch to his own +1.00 D sphere glasses and work through all the activities. The determination of +2.00 D spheres was done empirically; it would ease the task for him but would not make it too easy. In addition, a pair of +2.00 D spheres was available, so it was convenient to try them out with the patient while he was in the office and could be observed. Observations confirmed projections.

VISIT 4 (TWO WEEKS LATER)

Patient reports progress, but he has not yet been able to complete procedure 8 while wearing his own glasses; he can complete all the activities when wearing +2.00 D spheres (OU).

Re-administration of placement tests corroborates patient's report. He cannot yet achieve the goals of level II while wearing his own glasses.

A new procedure (4) is dispensed to patient along with a Variable-Mirror Stereoscope. It would have been acceptable to continue the patient on the procedure that was dispensed at the previous visit, but a new procedure was introduced because innovation inspires motivation.

VISIT 5 (TWO WEEKS LATER)

Patient reports satisfactory completion of procedure 4 while wearing his own glasses. Symptoms persist.

Re-administration of placement tests corroborates patient's report. He is able to achieve the goals of levels II and III; however, he cannot yet demonstrate the abilities called for by the level IV goal.

A new procedure (3-I, 3-II, and 3-III) is dispensed to patient along with the reassurance that he has made good progress and is close to completion of this aspect of the therapy program. He is also cautioned that this new procedure is lengthy and demanding; he is not to become discouraged if progress slows a bit. (For an explanation of why we typically select procedure 3 (I, II, and III) to complete a vergence infacility case, see p. 15.)

VISIT 6 (TWO WEEKS LATER)

Patient reports progress. His log shows that he has completed procedure 3-I, but not procedure 3-II; he has yet to try procedure 3-III. Symptoms have begun to diminish.

Re-administration of placement tests corroborates patient's report. He needs more time with procedure 3-II. He is advised to continue as is, and if he completes part III of procedure 3 before his next visit, he is to work through the entire procedure again, this time without his glasses. (This information was also entered into the special-instructions section of the printed handout he took home.)

VISIT 7 (TWO WEEKS LATER)

Patient reports successful completion of procedure 3-III, even when not wearing his glasses. Symptoms have disappeared.

Re-administration of placement tests shows successful completion of level IV. Patient is advised to continue to practice final activities daily, a few minutes at a time, until his next visit, about three months hence.

VISIT 8 (THREE MONTHS LATER)

Patient reports that he is symptom-free. He is able to read comfortably, even without his glasses; however, he does like to wear his glasses when he settles down to prolonged near-point tasks. He "sees clearly" either way, with and without his glasses, but just "feels better" if he wears his glasses on these occasions.

Examination reveals no significant change in phorias, but there is major improvement in fusional reserves and vergence facility at distance and near. (Not by coincidence, his accommodation facility has also improved markedly. Had it not, we would have prescribed additional therapy for this. Patient had been forewarned of this possibility and was now informed that it was not needed.) Patient is advised to continue practicing the final activity once a week until he returns for his annual re-examination. Case successfully completed.

CHAPTER 3

Accommodation Infacility

Accommodation infacility falls into the same general category as does vergence infacility. It represents a less-than-satisfactory capacity to adapt easily and rapidly to different demands on the accommodative system, even though the patient's visual acuity, refractive status, and binocular status are adequate. Traditionally, the optometrist comes close to assessing this with tests of positive and negative relative accommodation. These are well-established, useful tests, but they fail to take *facility* into account (facility is the patient's ability to adapt quickly and easily to abrupt changes in accommodation demands while vergence is held constant).

IDENTIFICATION

Signs and Symptoms

These assume that the patient has been wearing whatever lenses he needs to compensate fully for any existing ametropia. Not all of the following are necessarily experienced or displayed by all patients.

1. Discomfort (ocular pain, headaches, eyestrain, etc.) during or following prolonged visual activity
2. Avoidance of close work
3. Periodic blur at all fixation distances, especially when shifting from sustained near work to a far-point target
4. Reduced amplitude of accommodation

5. Reduced positive or negative relative accommodation ranges
6. Inadequate adaptation to abrupt changes in accommodation demands, especially when vergence posture is held constant

Prevalence

High in all pre-presbyopic age groups.

Screening Tests

To be conducted with patient wearing whatever lenses needed to compensate fully for existing ametropia.

Accommodation Facility at Distance

1. Patient fixates on a vertical row of small but legible letters (about 20/20 to 20/30) located 6 meters away. Examiner makes certain that the patient sees the letters singly and clearly.

2. Hold a pair of −2.00 D spheres before the patient's eyes and say, *"Tell me as soon as you are able to see these letters clearly; also, make sure you keep them single."* (Lenses may be from trial case and held in the examiner's hand, or they may be mounted in a so-called flipper frame.)

3. When, and if, the print clears and is single, remove the −2.00 D spheres, once more requesting that the patient report as soon as he again sees a single line of clear print. With young patients, it is advisable to validate their responses by having them read the letters; hence, the fixation target should be changed from time to time to eliminate the possibility of the patient's simply remembering what he saw previously.

4. As soon as the patient reports seeing the line singly and clearly without the lenses, re-introduce them, repeating step 2. Continue in this way until the patient has successfully accomplished three cycles, or until 30 seconds have elapsed, whichever occurs first. A cycle consists of letters clear and single through lenses, then clear and single when lenses are removed. Consider three cycles within 30 seconds to be satisfactory (passing) performance (see criteria below).

5. If the patient satisfies criterion (i.e., accomplishes three cycles within 30 seconds), test accommodation facility at near point (see below).

6. If the patient does not satisfy criterion (i.e., if he cannot successfully overcome the −2.00 D spheres), reduce lens power in 0.50 D increments and repeat procedure until he is able to execute three cycles within 30 seconds. Then, in order to rule out the possibility that he may simply have been a bit slow in understanding what he was to do, continue testing as you increase lens power in 0.50 D increments until threshold is determined. Record that lens power. For example, if initially the patient could not see clearly through the −2.00 D or −1.50 D but could adapt to the −1.00 D, then re-test with −1.50 D. If he

now is able to pass this level, go up again to the −2.00 D, and if he once again cannot accomplish three cycles with that power within 30 seconds, record threshold at −1.50 D, and go on to test accommodation facility at near.

Accommodation Facility at Near

1. Repeat the procedure described above, this time using small letters held at 40 cm. Also, because it is near point, probe the patient's facility at both activating and inhibiting accommodation with vergence held constant. Start with −2.00 D spheres (OU), as was just described for far-point testing. Remember, it is advisable to ensure the validity of a young patient's responses by having him actually read what he reports seeing clearly.

2. Once testing has been completed with the minus to plano cycle, administer the same type of tests with plus lenses, beginning with +2.00 D spheres.

Performance Criteria

These have been established arbitrarily but appear to be clinically valid. Consider accomplishment of the following to be satisfactory:

AT FAR	Plano to −2.00*
AT NEAR	Plano to +2.00*
	Plano to −2.00*

Just as with vergence infacility, if the optometrist believes that the patient does manifest accommodation infacility despite having passed the screening test or, vice versa, that the patient does not manifest accommodation infacility despite the screening test outcomes, professional judgment should prevail. In general, however, the criteria stated above will discriminate accurately between those patients who should and should not have clinical treatment.

TREATMENT

Factors the Optometrist Should Consider

Prognosis for Remediation Through Vision Therapy. Very favorable, especially in those cases where the patient demonstrates satisfactory stereopsis and a normal amplitude of accommodation.

Alternative Treatment Options

Reassurance The effects of leaving well enough alone in the management of accommodation infacility may not be significantly detrimental, but neither is it very helpful. The condition rarely deteriorates into a worse condition, but it is unlikely that the patient's symptoms will disappear. Hence, this is not the treatment of choice.

---

* Three cycles within 30 seconds

Referral There is rarely any need for consultation in these cases once the possibility of pathology has been ruled out.

Compensation If the patient does not display the intellectual, physiological, or motivational traits that are needed to benefit from vision therapy, consider prescribing compensatory lenses (i.e., additional plus power for near work; in bifocal form, if necessary) to reduce some of the stress he faces when engaging in demanding near-point visual activities. This will enable the patient to perform more comfortably despite the functional deficit, even though it will not eliminate the problem. How much lens power? That will vary with the case, but as a rule of thumb, use enough power to put into balance the relationship between the patient's positive (minus-to-blur) and negative (plus-to-blur) relative accommodation.

Factors the Patient Should Consider

Probable Outcome of Treatment. An improved capacity to engage comfortably in sustained near-point visual activities.

Consequences if Recommendations Are Not Followed. A lack of compliance will probably result in continuation of present symptoms and, perhaps, the need for compensatory lenses. It is not likely to result in a serious vision problem beyond the functional deficits.

Patient's Obligations. The patient will be required to devote about 10 to 15 minutes to prescribed remedial activities daily for approximately three to four weeks; this will be followed by two months or so of maintenance activities that will require about 1 to 2 minutes per day.

Number and Frequency of Office Visits. Patient should anticipate from four to six visits, depending on the level at which therapy begins and the rate at which he progresses. More specifically, if the patient places in level I (see below), successful treatment of accommodation infacility, on average, requires approximately six office visits. If the patient places in level II or higher, approximately two fewer office visits will be needed.

Implementation of Vision Therapy

Steps to be taken once the patient accepts the recommendation for vision therapy:

1. Schedule Patient for a Second Visit. At that visit, the office assistant will carry out the sequence of procedures described in chapter 1 (pp. 1–4), commencing with placement testing.

2. Placement Testing. Levels and goals, organized in descending order of difficulty (see also Table 3.1).

TABLE 3.1 Accommodation Facility Treatment Goals

	Lens powers, D	
Level	**Far**	**Near**
IV	plano to −2.50	−2.50 to +2.00
III	plano to −2.00	−2.50 to +1.50
II	plano to −1.00	−1.50 to +1.00
I	plano to −0.50	−1.00 to +0.50

Note: Rate = 60 cycles within 5 minutes. At far, a cycle comprises from plano to minus to plano; at near, from minus to plus to minus.

LEVEL IV

This is the final goal. Patient is able to clear and keep single a row of small vertical letters, executing accommodation jumps as follows:

AT FAR Plano to −2.50 D*
AT NEAR −2.50 D to +2.00 D*

Notice that these criteria are much more demanding than those of the screening test. Far-point criterion now calls for a 2.50-D, near-point, for a 4.50-Diopter accommodation jump, as compared with the 2.00-D adjustments of the screening test. The rationale for this is stated in chapter 1, pp. 2–3.

LEVEL III

AT FAR Plano to −2.00 D*
AT NEAR −2.50 D to +1.50 D*

LEVEL II

AT FAR Plano to −1.00 D*
AT NEAR −1.50 to +1.00 D*

LEVEL I

AT FAR Plano to −0.50 D*
AT NEAR −1.00 D to +0.50 D*

3. Patient's Performance. During placement testing, pay special attention to differences in performance the patient may display as a function of:

Fixation distance Some patients have much more difficulty exercising accommo-

* Sixty cycles within 5 minutes. For one cycle at far, start with no lenses, then introduce the minus lenses, then back to no lenses; at near, start with the minus lenses, then replace these with the plus lenses, then back to the minus lenses.

dation facility at distance than at near; others, vice versa. If there is a marked difference, therapy should begin at the fixation distance that presents the least difficulties. If no major difference is observed, then start where it is most convenient.

4. Select Procedure. Select appropriate procedure(s) from Table 3.2, keeping in mind the relative difficulty of near versus far fixation distance discussed above. Locate the procedure and photocopy it.*

5. Amend Procedure. Amend the procedure (in the special-instructions section of the handout) to make it more or less demanding, in accord with the patient's needs and the treatment goals. For example, a patient who has difficulty only in activating accommodation (i.e., adapting efficiently to minus spheres) is likely to have relatively less difficulty if he wears some base-out prism at the same time; the innervational link between convergence and accommodation will provide additional support. A similar link exists, of course, between base-in prism and the inhibition of accommodation. Therefore, it might serve the patient well to provide him with prisms in the form of training glasses that he wears while engaged in his therapy—compensating prisms if support is the goal, anti-compensating prisms if the goal is to increase the difficulty of the task (i.e., in the latter case, base-in prism to be worn while attempting to activate accommodation; base-out, while inhibiting accommodation).

6. Postplacement Testing. Continue with the postplacement testing sequence described in chapter 1 (pp. 1–4).

TABLE 3.2 Accommodation Facility Procedures

			This procedure is appropriate if the patient is to start therapy at		
Procedure	**Apparatus**	**Targets**	**Far**	**Near**	**Prerequisites**[a]
22	Minus lenses	Wall chart (newspaper)	X		B or D
23	Minus lenses; plus lenses	Vectogram 9		X	A
24	Minus lenses; plus lenses; nonvariable tranaglyph; red-green filters	Any nonvariable tranaglyph		X	A

[a] Prerequisites: A = third-degree fusion (i.e., stereopsis) at near; B = third-degree fusion at far; C = second-degree fusion (i.e., single, simultaneous, binocular vision) at near; D = second-degree fusion at far.

* Some patients manifest both vergence and accommodation infacility. For suggested procedures in such cases, see Table 3.2 and Procedures Manual.

CASE REPORTS

Patient 3.1

VISIT 1

Patient is a 20-year-old student. He has never worn glasses, although he has had previous eye examinations because of recurring asthenopic symptoms.

Chief Complaints Discomfort at extended close work; early onset of fatigue; print blurs upon extended reading; distance vision becomes blurred after prolonged reading.

Salient Clinical Data *Health status:* No evidence of pathology

Visual acuity: 20/20 each eye at distance and near

Refractive status: Emmetropia

Binocular status

AT FAR 1 PD exophoria
Stereoacuity: 1 min of arc
Accommodation facility: Fails screening test; does not adapt successfully to −2.00 D spheres (OU); is able to deal with −1.00 D spheres

AT NEAR 12 PD exophoria
Stereoacuity: 40 sec of arc
Near-point convergence: 11 in
Accommodation facility: Fails screening test; cannot adapt to minus lenses stronger than −1.00 D (OU); adapts satisfactorily to +2.00 D (OU)

All else within normal limits.

Conclusion Patient's symptoms probably derive from accommodation infacility.

Prescription Patient advised that his problem can be successfully treated two ways: (1) by wearing glasses that provide plus power for near work, and (2) by engaging in vision therapy, which would probably free him from the need for glasses. Patient selects the second option and is scheduled for second visit.

VISIT 2 (FOUR DAYS LATER)

Placement Testing Patient fails level I goals; hence he is placed in level I; therapy begins at this level. Procedure 22 is selected, photocopied, and dispensed to the patient along with two pairs of minus lenses: −1.50 D and −2.50 D.

The patient did not seem to have more difficulty at a given fixation distance, so this factor did not influence the decision regarding procedure. The procedure he was assigned stressed far-point function; it could just as easily have been one that required near-point fixation.

VISIT 3 (TWO WEEKS LATER)

Patient reports, and his daily log shows, satisfactory completion of procedure 22. Symptoms persist; in fact, they may be worse.

Re-administration of placement tests indicates that patient is now able to demonstrate the goals of levels I and II, but not of level III. Patient is assured that progress is being made.

Procedure 23 selected from Table 3.2, photocopied, and dispensed to the patient along with the appropriate pairs of plus lenses. Patient is advised to continue with the final activity of procedure 22 but to spend some time on procedure 23 as well (this procedure calls for near-point adaptations).

VISIT 4 (TWO WEEKS LATER)

Patient reports satisfactory completion of procedure 23. Symptoms have diminished; patient is able to read for longer periods without experiencing discomfort; print does not blur as often as before.

Re-administration of placement tests corroborates patient's report. He accomplishes the goals of level III.

A new procedure (24) is dispensed to patient, this one involving the use of plus and minus lenses in conjunction with a nonvariable-disparity tranaglyph. (Here we ask the patient to activate and inhibit accommodation while at the same time, but not necessarily in synchrony, activating and inhibiting convergence.)

VISIT 5 (TWO WEEKS LATER)

Patient reports satisfactory completion of procedure 24. Symptoms have disappeared for the most part; they manifest only when patient is exceptionally fatigued.

Re-administration of placement tests corroborates patient's report. He is able to achieve the goal of level IV with relative ease. All that remains is for the patient to continue to practice this final goal daily for the next two to four months. Patient is advised accordingly.

VISIT 6 (FOUR MONTHS LATER)

Patient has complied with instructions; has practiced final activity of procedure 24 daily for the past few months. Patient is symptom-free.

Re-administration of placement tests indicates that patient has acquired excellent accommodation facility at both distance and near.

Patient is advised to continue to practice final activity regularly—about once a week—until he returns for his annual visit. Case successfully completed.

CHAPTER 4

Intermittent Strabismus

The term *intermittent strabismus* as it is used in this chapter means that the patient displays two distinctly different binocular states during a given time span. At some times, he manifests strabismus; at other times, normal binocular alignment in at least one direction of gaze, which can be documented by better than 100 sec of arc stereoacuity at 6m and/or 60 sec of arc at 40 cm. These qualifications are critical in the context of this chapter. There are patients whose binocular status changes during the course of a day, from apparent alignment to very obvious misalignment, yet at no time are they able to display the above-cited stereoacuities. Such patients will not respond to vision therapy in the way this chapter describes; the information presented here is not applicable to them. For all practical purposes, they should be treated as constant strabismics. (For more discussion regarding this type of case, see chapter 6.)

IDENTIFICATION

Signs and Symptoms

These assume that the patient has been wearing whatever lenses he needs to compensate fully for any existing ametropia. Not all of the following are necessarily displayed or experienced by all patients.

1. Unstable binocularity and occasional diplopia attributable, in some cases, to a specific fixation distance; in others, to a specific direction of gaze, to fatigue, etc. (Diplopia is more common among intermittent esotropes than among intermittent exotropes.)

2. Significant heterophoria at one or more fixation distances, sometimes not apparent until the patient is fatigued or unless the phoria is measured after a relatively long period of prism- or occluder-induced disassociation. At those times, in fact, it is not uncommon to observe the heterophoria change to a heterotropia.

3. Reduced positive or negative fusional vergence ranges, at least at one fixation distance (i.e., far or near).

4. Inadequate vergence facility.

5. Some discomfort (headaches, eyestrain, etc.) during or following prolonged visual activity.

Prevalence

Manifested by approximately 2 to 3 percent of the population.

Screening Tests

To be conducted with patient wearing whatever lenses he needs to compensate fully for existing ametropia.

1. Unilateral cover tests, using both refined and crude fixation targets (e.g., a row of small letters, and again with a diffuse light source) held in the various positions of gaze at distance and at near. There are some patients who display unique (usually congenital) conditions wherein strabismus manifests in one position of gaze only and is caused by nerve or muscle paresis or an anatomical anomaly of some sort, (e.g., overactive superior or inferior oblique extraocular muscle, Brown's tendon sheath syndrome, Duane's syndrome). It is important to identify these conditions, explain them to the patient, and to recognize that they very rarely, if ever, respond to vision therapy. Most often, they are better treated by reassurance.

2. In some cases, it is difficult to differentiate between intermittent strabismus and a high heterophoria. It often depends upon the time of day that the patient is examined and other related factors (e.g., patient's fatigue state). Indeed, the patient who is diagnosed as manifesting intermittent strabismus in the late afternoon may very well have been diagnosed as having a vergence infacility problem had he been examined in the morning. It is a matter of threshold. Hence, if the unilateral cover test, routinely administered, does not reveal a problem, yet there is reason to suspect intermittent strabismus, the alternating cover and vergence facility screening tests should be administered or re-administered toward the end of the examination, when the patient is fatigued. (There is no practical reason to make this distinction; the treatment is the same for both conditions.)

3. There are instances when intermittent strabismus is elicited only if the patient fixates on a finely detailed (accommodation-demanding) stimulus that is held very close to his eyes. This situation—assuming that any existing ametropia is fully corrected—is usually caused by a high AC/A which may be apparent in other parts of the examination as well (e.g., esophoria that is significantly greater at near than at far). (See case report patient 4.3, p. 40.)

TREATMENT

Factors the Optometrist Should Consider

Prognosis for Remediation Through Vision Therapy. Favorable, *if* the patient meets the stereoacuity criteria defined in the introductory statements of this chapter.

Alternative Treatment Options

Reassurance Benign neglect of intermittent strabismus may or may not be detrimental, depending upon the nature of the deviation and the age of the patient. If ignored, intermittent esotropia in very young children often changes to constant esotropia. Intermittent exotropia tends to remain unchanged during those same early years; it usually does not get worse, but neither does it disappear. Hence, it is not wise to ignore the problem except in the cases of very young children with intermittent exotropia—children who are not yet sufficiently mature to benefit from vision therapy. In those cases, the decision about whether to reassure or to recommend lenses as interim treatment depends upon the frequency of the strabismus and the anxiety levels of the child's parents. If the child does not manifest strabismus more than about 20 percent of his waking hours, or if the child's parents are not overly anxious about doing nothing, then reassurance and regular monitoring of the case is the preferred treatment. If, on the other hand, the strabismus manifests more often than about 20 percent of the child's waking hours, or if the child's parents have difficulty managing their emotions in respect to the child's condition (and do not overlook the fact that they also have to cope with the anxieties of and pressures from other family members at the same time), then by all means consider interim (lens) treatment, at least until the child reaches the age when it is reasonable to institute a vision therapy regimen.

Referral There rarely is any need for consultation in these cases once the possibility of pathology has been ruled out. Intermittent strabismus is sometimes difficult to explain, but it is not difficult to diagnose and treat. It is well within the scope of the primary-care optometrist.

Compensation If the patient does not display the intellectual, physiological, or motivational traits needed to profit from vision therapy (see p. iii and Reassurance, above), consider the use of compensatory prisms (e.g., base-out for intermittent esotropes; base-in for intermittent exotropes). How much prism power? That will vary with the case, but in general, use enough prism to put the patient's phorias into balance with his fusional vergence reserves, enough so that he is able to maintain alignment without excessive effort.

Compensatory spheres should also be considered, especially for the patient with an unusually high AC/A ratio who manifests intermittent esotropia at near fixation only. Plus lenses for near only, in bifocal form, will help regardless of the patient's distance refractive status (i.e., they may be emmetropes, hyperopes, or, rarely, myopes). Compensatory spheres may also be useful in the intermittent exotrope–anxious parent situation described above. Minus lenses beyond what is called for by the patient's refractive status are likely to help him maintain bifoveal alignment. How much plus or minus power? Enough to make it possible for the patient to maintain alignment, or close to it, during the unilateral cover test.

Neither of these two approaches—prisms and plus or minus spheres as described here—should be viewed as remedial. They will not alter the underlying condition; they are simply methods for facilitating bifoveal alignment. Most patients will continue to manifest intermittent strabismus once the lenses have been abandoned. More than this is needed to alter the underlying clinical picture.

Factors the Patient Should Consider

Probable Outcome of Treatment. The patient will report fewer episodes of strabismus and faster recovery when it does manifest. Ultimately it will not manifest at all. (It is probably wise to inform the patient that during treatment there is not likely to be a significant change in the magnitude of the deviation when his eyes are in their strabismic posture; a 25 PD intermittent exotrope will continue to be a 25 PD intermittent exotrope when his strabismus manifests.)

Consequences If Recommendations Are Not Followed. A lack of compliance will probably result in the continuation of present signs and symptoms. It is not likely to result in a worsened visual status except in cases of young children with intermittent esotropia. If left unattended, their condition often deteriorates to constant esotropia.

Patient's Obligations. The patient will be required to engage in about 20 to 30 minutes of prescribed remedial activities daily for approximately four to eight weeks. This will be followed by six to nine months of maintenance activities that will require a few minutes per day. (As a rule, anticipate that the intermittent esotrope will need a little more time than the intermittent exotrope.)

Number and Frequency of Office Visits. The patient should anticipate between 9 and 12 visits, depending upon the level at which therapy begins and the rate at which he progresses. More specifically, if the patient places in level I, successful treatment of intermittent strabismus, on average, requires from 9 to 12 office visits. If the patient places in level II or higher, two or three fewer office visits will be needed.

Implementation of Vision Therapy

Steps to be taken once the patient accepts the recommendation for vision therapy:

1. Schedule Patient for a Second Visit. At that visit, the office assistant will carry out the sequence of procedures described in chapter 1, commencing with placement testing (see pp. 1–4.)

2. Placement Testing. Levels and goals, organized in descending order of difficulty.

LEVEL IV

This is the final goal. Patient is able to execute fusional vergence jumps as follows:

AT FAR From 6 PD base in *to* 12 PD base out, and vice versa,* *and*
AT NEAR From 12 PD base in *to* 14 PD base out, and vice versa*

The preceding goal may sound familiar, and with good reason: it is identical to the final goal in the vergence infacility sequence described in chapter 2. It is used here, as well, because there is no major difference between treating a patient with intermittent strabismus and one with vergence infacility except that the former will probably require some additional support to get started in the vision therapy sequence. The sequence itself remains the same. Hence, rather than repeat the sequence of subordinate goals and procedures already listed in chapter 2 (Tables 2.1 and 2.2), the reader is referred to that chapter but cautioned, also, to pay close attention to the directives stated immediately below.

3. Patient's Performance. During placement testing, pay special attention to differences in performance the patient may display as a function of

Compensatory lenses Some intermittent strabismics need compensatory lenses to get started in vision therapy procedures. For example, intermittent esotropes will often get off to a better start if they are given extra plus spheres in bifocal form for near fixation (see case report of patient 4.3, below). In some cases, the effect may be further enhanced by providing some base-out prisms as well. Conversely, intermittent exotropes often have less difficulty getting started in a procedure if they are supplied with minus lenses or base-in prisms. If this type of support appears to be called for, it should be supplied, then withdrawn as the patient makes progress and demonstrates that the support is no longer needed.

Direction of the vergence adaptation Some patients have much more difficulty with base-out prism demands than they do with base-in prism; others, vice versa. If there is a marked difference, take it into account when tailoring the initial therapy activities. For example, the intermittent esotrope is likely to have a more difficult time with base-in demand conditions; the intermittent exotrope, with base-out demand conditions. If it appears that this factor is sufficient to impede initial progress, start the patient with the condition that presents the least obstacle and work toward the opposite condition. (There are exceptions: some intermittent exotropes manifest their binocular instability only at far-point fixation; at near they display esophoria. Such patients may therefore get off to a better start if their initial vision therapy activities present a moderate base-out demand at near.)

---

* Sixty cycles within 5 minutes. For one cycle, start with fusion and clarity through base-in prisms (loose, hand-held, or mounted in flippers); then fusion and clarity through base-out prisms; then again through base-in. Test at far, then at near.

Fixation distance For some patients with intermittent strabismus, maintaining bifoveal alignment at distance is much more difficult than maintaining it at near; for others, vice versa. If there is a marked difference, therapy should begin at the fixation distance that presents the least difficulty. If no major difference is observed, then start where it is most convenient.

4. Select Procedure. Select appropriate procedure(s) from Table 2.2 (p. 12), keeping in mind the three factors mentioned above (i.e., relative effects of compensatory lenses, direction of vergence adaptation, and fixation distance). Locate the procedure in the Procedures Manual and photocopy it.

5. Amend Procedure. Amend the procedure in the special-instructions section of the printed handout to make it more or less demanding, in accord with the patient's needs and the treatment goals. The remarks in chapter 2 regarding this step pertain here as well (see p. 11).

6. Postplacement Testing. Continue with the postplacement testing sequence as described in chapter 1 (see pp. 1–4).

CASE REPORTS

Patient 4.1—Divergence Excess

VISIT 1

Patient is a 10-year-old with a long history of intermittent exotropia. Condition first manifested when he was 2 years old. Essentially unchanged since that time. No other ocular complaints.

Chief Complaints

Intermittent exotropia that usually manifests when patient is tired and/or in a daydreamlike posture before the TV set.

Salient Clinical Data

Health status: No evidence of pathology
Visual acuity: 20/20 each eye at distance and near
Refractive status: Emmetropia
Binocular status

AT FAR

12 PD exophoria without lenses (orthophoria when measured while patient fixates through −2.00 D spheres. (OU))
Stereoacuity: 1 min of arc (when eyes are in alignment)
Vergence facility: Fails, is unable to adapt to more than 6 PD base out.

AT NEAR 6 PD exophoria
Stereoacuity: 40 sec of arc (when eyes are in alignment)
Near-point convergence: 4 cm
Vergence facility: Adapts successfully to 12 PD base in and 14 PD base out. Hence, he passes this part of the screening test.

All else within normal limits.

Conclusion Intermittent exotropia that manifests upon distance fixation (i.e., divergence excess).

Prescription Either compensatory lenses (base-in prisms) for full-time wear or vision therapy. The latter is recommended. Patient accepts recommendation and is scheduled for second visit.

VISIT 2 (ONE WEEK LATER)

Placement Testing Placement testing always starts with level I goals. Patient fails level I. He has no difficulty adapting to the base-in or base-out prisms but is unable to appreciate physiological diplopia. Therefore, placement is in level I; therapy begins at that level.

Procedure 19 (physiological diplopia) is selected, photocopied, and dispensed to the patient with full explanation of how to engage in the activity at home.

VISIT 3 (ONE WEEK LATER)

Patient reports satisfactory completion of procedure 19 but no change in visual condition.

Re-administration of placement tests indicates that patient now meets the goals of level I, but not level II. (This seems to contradict the vergence facility data obtained during the second visit, but, in fact, it does not. As is the case with many intermittent exotropes, the patient is able to adapt to base-out prism when it is introduced from the no-prism condition, but not when it replaces base-in prism; also, the patient is not able to sustain the vergence jumps for as long as the criteria require.) Patient is assured that progress is being made.

Procedure 9 is selected from Table 2.2, photocopied, and dispensed to the patient along with the minitranaglyphs. (The procedure could have been any of those listed in Table 2.2. Procedure 9 was selected primarily because the patient is more adept at near point than at far point and because there was a minitranaglyph available in the office that day.)

VISIT 4 (TWO WEEKS LATER)

Patient reports progress but not completion of procedure 9; that is, he cannot yet accomplish the jumps called for by the instructions.

Re-administration of placement tests corroborates patient's report. He cannot achieve the goals of level II because of an inability to execute the vergence jumps.

A new procedure (3-I) is dispensed to patient along with a set of near-point eccentric rectangle targets.

It would have been equally acceptable to continue the patient with the procedure that was dispensed at the previous visit. The reason for introducing a new procedure was that innovation generates motivation; in addition, this new procedure was one that he can continue to use throughout the treatment program. (For an explanation of why we usually select procedure 3 in these cases, see p. 15.)

VISIT 5 (TWO WEEKS LATER)

Patient reports satisfactory completion of procedure 3-I.

Re-administration of placement tests corroborates patient's report. He is able to achieve the goal of level II with relative ease; however, he is not yet able to demonstrate the abilities called for by the level III goal.

Patient is advised to continue practicing the final activity of procedure 3-I, and a new procedure (3-II) is added to the regimen.

VISIT 6 (TWO WEEKS LATER)

Patient reports progress with procedures 3-I and 3-II but not complete facility. His parents also report that they have noticed a significant reduction in the incidence of their son's strabismus.

Re-administration of placement tests corroborates patient's report. He is able to demonstrate the goal of level III without difficulty. Patient is advised accordingly, and procedure 3-III is added to this regimen.

VISIT 7 (TWO WEEKS LATER)

Patient has complied with instructions; he is able to carry out all the activities of procedures 3-I and 3-II. He still fatigues when attempting to do the final activity of procedure 3-III; he rarely is able to get through it successfully.

Re-administration of placement tests indicates that patient has progressed significantly but cannot yet demonstrate mastery of the final (level IV) goals of the treatment program.

Patient is advised to continue to practice final activity of procedure 3-III regularly.

VISIT 8 (TWO WEEKS LATER)

Patient reports continued progress; he is now able to do the final steps of procedure 3-III. His parents note continued improvement in the strabismus; it rarely manifests.

Re-administration of placement tests indicates that patient can meet the requirements of level IV. All that remains is for the patient to practice this final activity daily for the next three to four months.

VISIT 9 (THREE MONTHS LATER)

Patient reports compliance with instructions. He has practiced his final activities regularly and has become very adept at them.

Assessment confirms that report. Patient is able to execute vergence jumps at far and near in excess of what is called for in the goals of level IV. Cover test continues to elicit an intermittent exotropia but with two significant differences when compared with patient's performance at pretraining visits: (1) It is more difficult to provoke the strabismus; short-term occlusion will not do it; the occluder has to be held in place for a prolonged period before the strabismus is observed (i.e., about 15 to 20 seconds). (2) the exotropic eye returns to alignment almost instantaneously, whereas previously the patient had to "think about it for a second or two" before the eye would align; in other words, it now looks more like a case of heterophoria rather than heterotropia.

Patient is advised to continue to practice final activity of procedure 3-III for a few minutes once each week for the next six months. (We suggested that patient select a time during the week when he regularly does something, for instance, when he is getting ready to go to church.

VISIT 10 (SIX MONTHS LATER)

Patient reports compliance with recommendations. His parents report that they have not observed the exotropia for well over the past three months.

Assessment reveals a continuation of the significant exophoria at far point, but the patient displays no difficulty in managing it. He has acquired excellent vergence facility.

Patient is advised to continue to check himself on some regular basis (i.e., go through the final exercise of his program once in a while). We anticipate that, over time, his heterophoria will diminish—at least to the extent that it is revealed with short-term occlusion. No treatment beyond that is needed.

Patient 4.2—Convergence Insufficiency

VISIT 1

Patient is a 9-year-old student.

Chief Complaints

Fatigue at close work; occasional diplopia at near; symptoms began about one year ago, have gotten worse. Never wore glasses; this is first eye examination. Parents report that the child has always been a good student but that his school performance has deteriorated recently. They are inclined to "blame this on his eyes."

Salient Clinical Data

Health status: No evidence of pathology
Visual acuity: 20/20 each eye at distance and near
Refractive status: (OU) +0.50 − 0.50 cx 180
Binocular status

AT FAR
Orthophoria
Stereoacuity: 1 min of arc
Vergence facility: Passes screening test
Accommodation facility: Passes screening tests

AT NEAR 10 PD exophoria
Stereoacuity: 40 sec of arc
Near point of convergence: 30 cm
Vergence facility: Fails, cannot adapt to more than 2 PD base out; does meet base-in criteria.
Accommodation facility: Fails, cannot clear through powers in excess of +1.00 D spheres (OU).

All else within normal limits.

Conclusion

Patient's symptoms are probably caused by inadequately compensated exophoria at near, which deteriorates to exotropia when he is fatigued.

Prescription

Patient advised that his condition may be treated one of two ways: (1) by wearing glasses (base-in prism) for near work, or (2) by engaging in vision therapy. Vision therapy is recommended and patient accepts this option.

Patient is scheduled for second visit.

VISIT 2 (ONE WEEK LATER)

Placement Testing

Decision was made to ignore accommodation infacility at placement testing—although certain relevant procedures will probably be included in the treatment regimen—because as patient develops the ability to cope with his convergence insufficiency, his accommodation facility will also improve.

Patient fails level I vergence facility goals (Table 2.1). He cannot adapt to the base-out prism requirements of that level, nor is he able to appreciate physiological diplopia.

Hence, placement is in level I; therapy begins at this level. Procedure 5 (Adult Base-Out Comfort Series) is selected, photocopied, and dispensed to the patient along with a Brewster stereoscope. (Procedure 5 was chosen because the patient displayed significantly more difficulty at near than at far fixation. Procedures 6 and 12 would also have satisfied this condition.) Procedure 21 is also prescribed. (Here, again, an alternative procedure, 19 or 20, would have been equally suitable.)

VISIT 3 (TWO WEEKS LATER)

History Update

Patient's daily log shows satisfactory completion of both training procedures. His symptoms persist.

Re-administration of placement tests indicates that patient is now able to meet the goals of level I but not level II. Patient is assured that progress is being made.

Procedure 8 is selected from Table 2.2, photocopied, and dispensed to the patient along with a minivectotrainer.

This procedure focuses on near-point facility. Not surprisingly, patient displayed some difficulty with this activity when it was dispensed. For this reason, the procedure was amended in the special-instructions section of the printed handout to incorporate the use of 6 D prisms, base-in [training glasses] until he was able to get through the activities without them. Patient was supplied with a lens holder and two 3 D prism lenses. It was not critical to supply exactly 6 D of prism; anything approximating that would have served equally well. The main concern was to give the patient enough prism to ease his way into the activities of the procedure.

VISIT 4 (TWO WEEKS LATER)

Patient reports progress, but he is not yet able to complete procedure 8 without the training glasses; he can complete it when he is using the prism.

Re-administration of placement tests corroborates patient's report. He cannot yet achieve the goals of level II without the training glasses.

Patient advised to continue with same procedure and to work toward being able to complete all of the activities without the aid of the training glasses. (It would have been acceptable to dispense a different procedure to the patient; however, he did not appear to be bored nor overly frustrated with what he had been doing; hence the decision to continue as is.)

VISIT 5 (TWO WEEKS LATER)

Patient reports satisfactory completion of procedure 8 without the aid of the training glasses. Symptoms persist.

Re-administration of placement tests corroborates patient's report. He is able to achieve the goals of level II with relative ease. However, he cannot meet the requirement of level III.

A new procedure (16) is dispensed to patient along with a Red-Green Stereo Trainer. He is assured that he is making progress. (Procedure 16 was selected at this point because it allows the patient to engage in distance, midrange, or near activities. The base-in prisms were put aside; they were no longer necessary.)

VISIT 6 (TWO WEEKS LATER)

Patient reports progress with his new procedure (16) but was not able to complete it. Symptoms have begun to ease.

Re-administration of placement tests corroborates patient's report. His near point of convergence is now 7 cm. Nonetheless, he needs more time with level III activities. He is given a new procedure (3-I) and a pair of near-point eccentric rectangle targets.

VISIT 7 (TWO WEEKS LATER)

Patient reports successful completion of procedure 3-I. He no longer experiences symptoms.

Re-administration of placement tests shows successful completion of level III.

Patient is given a new procedure (3-II) and a pair of far-point eccentric rectangle targets. In addition, he is advised to continue practicing the final activity of procedure

3-I, but now while wearing a pair of +1.00 D spheres. (Obviously, the inclusion of the +1.00 D spheres increased the difficulty of the task—something that the patient was ready for).

VISIT 8 (TWO WEEKS LATER)

Patient's daily log shows successful completion of procedure 3-II. His parents report that his school work has improved significantly and that he no longer complains about his eyes. They inquire about the need for further treatment.

Re-administration of placement tests shows that patient does not quite meet the criteria of level IV goals.

Parents are advised accordingly and urged to continue the treatment for a few more sessions. They agree. Child is instructed to continue with what he has been doing.

VISIT 9 (TWO WEEKS LATER)

Child reports completion of all the activities on the last procedure dispensed. He is not as motivated as he once was and is inclined to bring the treatment program to a stop.

Assessment indicates that patient's binocular status has reached a satisfactory level.

Patient is informed that training has reached the stage where all that is required is maintenance, short, daily sessions that will aid in making the newly learned skills habitual. He is given procedure 3-III and asked to do this daily for the next four months, then return for reassessment.

Patient agrees.

VISIT 10 (18 MONTHS LATER)

Patient returns, complaining of a recurrence of symptoms. (He did not keep his last appointment.) His parents state that he failed to follow through with the maintenance activities; he saw "no reason" to do it.

Reassessment reveals regression. The child's near point of convergence has receded to about 25 cm; his vergence facility is also substandard, well below what it was at his last visit.

Patient is advised to resume vision therapy, starting off where he left off the year before. (The feasibility of this suggestion was examined in the office before it was offered. It appeared to be a reasonable recommendation; he could get through the activity, although it was a struggle.) A follow-up visit was scheduled for one month hence.

VISIT 11 (ONE MONTH LATER)

Patient reports that he has complied with recommendation and that results have been significant; his eyes "feel much better."

Reassessment corroborates his observations.

Patient is advised to commence maintenance activities and to return in one month.

VISIT 12 (ONE MONTH LATER)

Patient reports compliance.

Reassessment indicates no need for additional treatment.

Patient is advised to continue maintenance activities for a few minutes daily for the next six months.

VISIT 13 (SIX MONTHS LATER)

Patient reports continued compliance.

Reassessment indicates successful completion of treatment.

Patient is advised to engage in maintenance activities on a once-per-week basis for the following year. Patient is also assured that, should he regress, it will be only a matter of a few days' effort to restore the binocular status to its present condition.

Patient 4.3—Convergence Excess

VISIT 1

Patient is a 5-year-old kindergarten student.

Chief Complaints

Parents report that child's eyes cross when he looks at something held close to his face. First noted about six months ago; discussed at that time with pediatrician who counseled them to wait a bit to see if he "grew out of it." Child has no complaints; however, he has not performed up to expectations in kindergarten; his teacher says that he is distractible and inattentive.

Salient Clinical Data

Health status: No evidence of pathology
Visual acuity: 20/20+ each eye at distance and near
Refractive status: (OU) plano
Binocular status

AT FAR
- Orthophoria
- Stereoacuity: 1 min of arc
- Vergence facility: Passes screening test
- Accommodation facility: Inconclusive

AT NEAR
- 6 PD esophoria
- Stereoacuity: 40 sec of arc
- Vergence facility: Fails, cannot adapt to more than 2 PD base in; meets base-out criteria.
- Near-point convergence: 25 cm (When fixation object is held closer than this, he manifests marked esotropia.)
- Accommodation facility: Fails minus lens component

All else within normal limits.

Conclusion

Patient's symptoms are probably attributable to esophoria at near in combination with a high AC/A ratio.

Prescription

Parents are advised that child's problem, considering his age, is best treated by wearing glasses that provide additional plus power for near. (It was explained to the parents that the patient's "pointing muscles" overreact when his "focussing muscles" go to work; see pp. 126–128.) Vision therapy is not recommended; the child is too young to benefit sufficiently from such an approach.

Recommendation is accepted. Lenses are prescribed—(OU) plano/+3.00 add—with segs set very high in lenses. This last factor is essential. Positioning the segs high in the lens will not bother the child; he is not very tall; the floor will not be all that blurred. And more to the point, unless the segs are positioned high, the child will not use them for close work. He is not a presbyope; he does not need the extra power to see clearly. He needs the extra power to relax accommodation and, in turn, the convergence that his high AC/A generates. Hence, the segs have to be positioned so that the child uses them for near simply because they are there and in the way. Child to return in about three months.

VISIT 2 (THREE MONTHS LATER)

Parents report that child has worn glasses without complaint. Esotropia very rarely manifests. School performance has improved.

Reassessment indicates that lenses are neutralizing the esophoria effectively. Child continues to manifest high esophoria at near without glasses, but this reduces to 1 PD exophoria through the plus-lens add.

Parents are advised that child should continue to wear glasses for at least the next year. Then the situation will be reconsidered.

VISIT 3 (ONE YEAR LATER)

Parents report that child has started to resist wearing his glasses. He is now in first grade, and in their opinion, he does not like the glasses because of social pressures. Child has not manifested any symptoms or other indications of the original condition. He is doing well in first grade.

Assessment reveals more or less the same situation that was documented at visit 1, with the distinct exception that he is not so prone to esotropia as he once was.

Prescription

Because of the child's negative attitude toward glasses, it was agreed that vision therapy should be given a try. We stressed that he was still quite young for such a regimen, but perhaps it was worth a trial.

Placement Tests

Child fails level I vergence facility goals (Table 2.1); he cannot appreciate physiological diplopia nor can he adapt to the base-in prisms at distance or near.

Procedures 19 and 10 (physiological diplopia and quoit vectograms, respectively) are dispensed. The latter is amended in the special-instructions section of the handout to take into account the child's need for plus spheres at near point; he is to do all near point activities while looking through the +3.00 add in his old glasses.

VISIT 4 (TWO WEEKS LATER)

Parents report that child has complied with instructions, has mastered the final activity of procedure 19, but not the final activity of procedure 10.

Re-administration of placement testing corroborates this. The child is now capable of recognizing physiological diplopia but cannot adapt efficiently to base-in prisms at near point.

Parents are advised to continue on with procedure 10 until the next visit.

VISIT 5 (TWO WEEKS LATER)

Child has followed instructions and has made headway with his exercises. Parents also comment that they no longer notice any manifestation of the esotropia, even when the child is not wearing his glasses.

Placement retesting shows that child has mastered level I goals; in fact, he also meets criteria of level II goals. On the strength of this, procedure 24 is dispensed along with a nonvariable-disparity tranaglyph, a lens holder, and appropriate plus and minus lenses. An appointment is made for two weeks hence. (Procedure 24 was selected because of the child's high AC/A ratio. Learning to adapt to abrupt changes in accommodation demands while holding vergence constant will be beneficial.) The handout is amended to advise that if the child completes the procedure before his next visit, he should go back to the beginning and work through it again, this time without his glasses.

VISIT 6 (TWO WEEKS LATER)

Child continues to comply. Parents report that he has not been able to get through all the activities of procedure 24 with his glasses. Obviously, then, he did not try to work through them without the glasses.

Re-administration of placement tests validates their report. Child remains in level III; he does not appear to have made much headway since last visit.

Parents are advised to continue with present procedure and return in two weeks.

VISIT 7 (TWO WEEKS LATER)

Child remains compliant; however, he has not made much progress in the procedure dispensed a couple of visits ago. In addition, his school work has started to deteriorate.

Re-administration of placement tests shows that child remains in level III, even when tested through his segs.

Parents are advised that another couple of weeks should determine whether he should keep on with the vision therapy, will improve any more at this time, or should simply continue to wear his glasses—at least for school work. Parents agree to continue vision therapy for at least two more weeks.

VISIT 8 (TWO WEEKS LATER)

Parents report no progress. Child has been wearing his glasses constantly while in school and seems to be doing better because of it.

Re-administration of placement tests shows no progress. Parents are advised that, although the child has benefitted from the vision therapy, he appears to have reached a ceiling, at least for the present.

Hence, vision therapy is stopped; child to wear glasses and return next year for reassessment and reconsideration of recommendations.

Parents agree.

VISIT 9 (ONE YEAR LATER)

Child has been wearing glasses in school and does not appear to be having any difficulties. Assessment indicates no change in visual status.

Recommendation Continue as is, at least for the next year or two. Then, reconsider treatment options.

VISIT 10 (ONE YEAR LATER)

Child stopped wearing his glasses about six months ago. At first, he seemed to get along quite well. Lately, however, he has begun complaining about blurred vision at distance. He is doing well in school.

Assessment reveals very slight myopia, both eyes.

Visual acuity without glasses: 20/30, each eye

Refractive status: (OU) −0.50 D spheres; 20/20 each eye

Binocular status without glasses

Satisfactory at distance (i.e., orthophoria, 1 min of arc stereoacuity, satisfactory vergence and accommodation facility)

Relatively satisfactory at near (i.e., 5 PD esophoria, 30 sec of arc stereoacuity, unsatisfactory vergence facility, fails base-in component

Binocular status with new lens prescription: esophoria at near increases to 9 PD

Prescription On the basis of these data, a new lens prescription is issued that compensates for the modest amount of myopia but also incorporates plus lens addition for near work: +2.50 D sphere add (OU). Vision therapy is deferred until the child matures a bit more, perhaps a year or two hence. Parents accept recommendation.

Case is not yet completed; child will be reexamined in about six months. If conditions are appropriate, vision therapy will be reinstituted, this in an attempt to reduce the child's dependence upon the plus lenses for near.

CHAPTER 5

Amblyopia

The term *amblyopia* in this context refers to reduced visual acuity that does not improve to 20/20 with compensatory lenses and is not attributable to anatomical anomalies or pathology. ("Reduced visual acuity" applies to as slight a reduction as 20/25.) Amblyopia is typically observed in patients who were deprived of detailed visual stimulation during their early years because of constant unilateral strabismus, anisometropia, significant bilateral ametropia, or an anatomical defect (e.g., congenital or early-acquired cataract, corneal opacity) that was not successfully treated during the child's first four to six (or so) years.

IDENTIFICATION

Signs and Symptoms

Reduced visual acuity, usually in one eye only (but can be bilateral), that can be attributed to one of the conditions cited above.

Prevalence

Manifested by approximately 2 to 2.5 percent of the general population.

Screening Tests

To be conducted with patient wearing whatever lenses he needs to compensate fully for existing ametropia.

Visual acuity The amblyopic patient is detected without special screening tests. His condition becomes apparent during the course of a routine vision evaluation.

TREATMENT

Factors the Optometrist Should Consider

Prognosis for Remediation Through Vision Therapy. This depends upon the cause of the amblyopia, the age at which that cause manifested, and the age when proper treatment was instituted. For example, prognosis is far more optimistic for the 2-year-old strabismic child whose eyes were in alignment until he was 18 months old, than for the 10-year-old who has displayed constant unilateral strabismus since birth and has never been treated. Similarly, the prognosis is much more optimistic for the anisometropic patient who has never worn glasses and is now 3 years old than it is for a child with the same refractive condition and treatment history who is now 8 years old.

Alternative Treatment Options

Reassurance There are three types of amblyopic patients who are best served by reassurance: (1) the patient who has already received appropriate treatment for unilateral amblyopia with little or no success; (2) the adult patient with unilateral strabismic or anisometropic amblyopia who, though never treated, is now well past the so-called critical period of vision development,* and though he may respond somewhat to treatment, he will not respond as well or as permanently as he would have when he was younger; and (3) the bilateral amblyope.

An example of the first type is the 10-year-old patient with congenital, unilateral strabismus who, when he was 4, constantly wore a patch over his "good" eye for a year and showed only limited improvement in acuity (i.e., obtained 20/70 fairly quickly but stopped there). There is no reason to think that better results will be obtained now that he is older, so long as it is certain that he complied with the treatment when he was younger.

A fairly common circumstance exemplifies the second type: a young-adult patient with unilateral amblyopia that is attributable to marked anisometropia, for example, (OD) Plano; (OS) +5.50 −3.75 cx 180. He received his first glasses at age 6 but rarely wore them. Glasses were tried again when he was 8, with the same results. He has had no other treatment. Such patients do sometimes respond to vision therapy; the visual acuity of the amblyopic eye improves a line or two but never to anything approximating the acuity of the other eye (see patient 5.1 in case reports). Some practitioners would propose the "spare-tire argument" in these situations and reason that even though the patient does not normally use the amblyopic eye unless compelled to by some artificial means (e.g., a patch), he may need to use it at some future date, given the always-existing possibility that some unfortunate circumstance may befall the good eye. Hence, he should be treated now, just in case. The argument is not false, but

*Just what the "critical period" is for humans has not yet been precisely determined. Most authorities tend to agree that it consists of the first four to six years of life, more or less. When the phase is used in this book, it refers to that definition.

TABLE 5.1 Patching Regimen

Age of patient, yrs	Patch on[a]	
	Good eye	Poor eye
Younger than 1	2 days	1 day
1–3	3 days	1 day
3–4	4 days	1 day
Older than 4	6 days	1 day

the accompanying implication is—that one should do something to improve the amblyopic eye now and not take the risk of putting off treatment until it is too late. The fact is that this patient, who is already past the developmental period, will respond the same to amblyopia treatment later as he does now, even if treatment is held off for many years. The potential for improvement that exists now will continue to exist so long as nothing alters the integrity of the visual system in the meantime (e.g., cataract, corneal scar, central nervous system lesion). Should the latter occur, it will, of course, alter the above-described optimistic outlook, but the same negative effects would also be suffered by the patient who did receive amblyopia treatment now. In other words, once the patient is past the critical period of vision development, the spare-tire argument is not valid.

An example of the third type is a patient with significant bilateral hyperopic astigmatism—for example, (OU) +5.00 −4.00 cx 150—who did not begin to wear glasses until age 6. There is very little that the optometrist can do for this type of amblyopia except to prescribe compensatory lenses as early as possible, relieve whatever anxieties there may be about the long-term implications of the condition (i.e., that it will not deteriorate further and that it will not ultimately cause blindness), and instruct the patient and his parents about the importance of early identification should others in the family have a similar condition.

Referral There is no need for consultation in the treatment of amblyopia once the possibility of pathology has been ruled out.

Compensation There are very few useful compensatory treatments for amblyopia. Obviously, the foremost of these is to provide the patient with whatever lenses he needs to obtain the best visual acuity possible under the circumstances. Beyond that, compensatory treatment consists of low-vision optical aids or special placement in school or work; for example, enrollment in a class for the visually handicapped if that is justified, or simply a seat closer to the front in a standard classroom. These approaches are rarely needed, however; the vast majority of amblyopes manifest the condition in one eye only, thereby eliminating the need for special treatment in school or work.

Factors the Patient Should Consider

Probable Outcome of Treatment. Improved eyesight in the amblyopic eye, although one cannot predict just what visual acuity will ultimately be obtained.

Consequences If Recommendations Are Not Followed. A lack of compliance will result, at best, in the continuation of the present signs and symptoms. If the patient is very young, neglect may result in further deterioration of visual acuity. Hence, the younger the patient, the more important it is to institute therapy at once.

Patient's Obligations. This depends upon the nature of the treatment, which, in turn, depends upon the patient's age and binocular status (see below). In all cases, it is impossible to predict how long treatment will go on. The only reasonable method is to begin therapy, assess outcomes on a regular (weekly, biweekly, or monthly) basis, and proceed accordingly.

If the patient is not binocular and only one eye is amblyopic, he will be required to wear a patch, perhaps constantly, perhaps only for a limited time each day (see below). He may also be assigned certain supplementary activities to be done while the patch is in place.

If the patient is binocular and only one eye is amblyopic, he will not need to wear a patch, but he will have to engage in 15 to 30 minutes of vision therapy activities daily.

Number and Frequency of Office Visits. If the only condition being treated is amblyopia—that is, if this treatment is not one step in a larger effort, such as the treatment of constant strabismus or a perceptual skills disorder—then the situation is best managed on a one-visit-at-a-time basis, with treatment stopping when improvement stops. Preschool children should be seen at least once every week or two; older children, about once a month. Ordinarily, three to six months of treatment provides as much of an effect as is going to be obtained. Hence, most patients should anticipate that between three and six visits will be required.

Implementation of Vision Therapy

The sequence of steps to be taken once the patient elects to accept the recommendation for vision therapy will vary, depending upon the binocular–not binocular dichotomy mentioned above.

1. If the Patient Is Not Binocular. If the patient is not binocular and only one eye is amblyopic, then a second visit is not required before initiating the therapy program. All the necessary information will have been acquired during the initial visit; namely, the patient's lens prescription, his best corrected visual acuity in each eye, his binocular status, and a determination of the accuracy of fixation in the amblyopic eye. (Eccentric fixation does not require a different treatment, but it is worth documenting to serve as a benchmark when attempting to assess the effects of the treatment.)

Patching therapy, therefore, should commence at the conclusion of the first visit.

with part-time or constant occlusion of the non-amblyopic eye. The decision for part-time or constant occlusion is usually made on the basis of such factors as:

The patient's age The younger the patient, the more susceptible the non-amblyopic eye is to detrimental effects from occlusion. In fact, occlusion can produce amblyopia in very young children. The best method for managing patching is to alternate the patch from one eye to the other on a regularly scheduled basis, thereby providing the better eye some visual stimulation, but not so much as to neutralize the effects of the treatment on the amblyopic eye. The guidelines shown in Table 5.1 have been found to be effective.

How the patient spends his day Preschool-aged children encounter fewer problems from full-time patching than do older patients. The elementary school–aged child, whose visual acuity in the amblyopic eye is very poor (e.g., 20/200) will not be able to comply with the therapy yet meet the requirements of his classroom. A part-time regimen will be more suitable for him, at least until school vacation commences. (Indeed, there is a fair amount of published evidence that indicates that part-time patching does have beneficial effects, that constant occlusion is not essential.)

Supplementary activities Patching therapy often appears to be more effective if the patient engages in specific (hand-eye) activities while the patch is in place. This is especially so if the patch is not worn full time. A variety of these activities are described in procedure 34 (see Table 5.2 and the Procedures Manual).

Once treatment has been prescribed, schedule the patient for a follow-up visit as suggested above and proceed with this format until visual acuity achieves asymptote—as documented by one or two follow-up visits where no improvement is observed.

Also as suggested above, if the patient displayed eccentric fixation at the onset of treatment, some on going monitoring may be worthwhile. This is not really an important factor, but may be interesting. (If an eccentric fixator commences to become more of a central fixator as a result of the treatment, it will be revealed by improvement in visual acuity. Hence, as assessment of the accuracy of fixation simply helps explain the improvement in visual acuity—nothing more.)

The patch The patch may take the form of a piece of cloth, nail polish, or translucent mending tape placed over the patient's spectacle lens, or a bandage taped directly over his eyelid. If the patch is to be worn constantly, the latter is preferred. There are a number of commercially produced occluders, including the Opticlude eye patch (MMM) and the Elastoplast Eye Occlusor. Your local pharmacist will be able to show you what is available. (Keep in mind that some patients are allergic to the adhesives on these occluders. In turn, some occluders are hypoallergenic.)

2. If the Patient Is Binocular. If the patient is binocular and only one eye is amblyopic, then a second visit to initiate the therapy program will be necessary, not to conduct placement testing but, rather, to explain to the patient the procedure(s) he is to

TABLE 5.2 Amblyopia Procedures

Procedure	Apparatus and targets	Patient is Binocular	Patient is Monocular	Prerequisites[a]
1	Aperture Rule	X		A
4	Variable-Mirror Stereoscope; stereoscopic targets	X		A or C
6	Brewster stereoscope; Children's Base-Out Stories	X		B
7	Brewster stereoscope; Children's Base-In Stories	X		B
8	Minivectograms; Polaroid filters	X		A, E
9	Minitranaglyphs; red-green filters	X		A, E
10	Variable-disparity vectotrainer; quoit	X		A, E
11	Nonvariable-disparity tranaglyph	X		A, E
12	Brewster stereoscope; Base-Out Storybook Cards	X		B
13	Brewster stereoscope; Base-In Storybook Cards	X		B
14	Variable-disparity vectotrainer; any variable-disparity vectograms (e.g., Topper)	X		A, E
15	Variable-disparity tranaglyphs; any variable-disparity tranaglyphs	X		A, E
16	Red-green stereo trainer; red-green filters	X	X	A, B
19	Brock string, pens, etc.	X	X	C, D
20	Near-far fixations; two targets	X	X	C, D
21	Phy-Dip Stick	X		C
24	Nonvariable tranaglyph; plus and minus lenses	X		A, E
28	Variable-mirror stereoscope/cheiroscope	X		A or C
29	Single-mirror stereoscope/cheiroscope	X		A or C
30	Brewster stereoscope/cheiroscope	X		B or D
31	Red-green bar reader and filters	X		A or C
32	Red pencil and red-green filters	X		A or C
33	Miscellaneous	X		B or D
34	Miscellaneous		X	None

[a] Prerequisites: A = third-degree fusion (i.e., stereopsis) at near; B = third-degree fusion at far; C = second-degree fusion at near; D = second-degree fusion at far; E = well-established awareness of physiological diplopia.

engage in at home. Occlusion is not recommended for this type of patient. Instead, he should engage in activities that stimulate the amblyopic eye while the non-amblyopic eye is open and functioning. Several of these activities are listed in Table 5.2.

The office assistant should photocopy and dispense one or more of these at that second visit.

Other remedial methods for treating amblyopia have been proposed over the years. These include pleoptics, watching a rotating disc of black and white stripes, wearing inverse prisms, "penalizing" the non-amblyopic eye with a drug, blurring the non-amblyopic eye with a high plus lens, wearing a red filter before one eye, and so on. Each has had its proponents; each has had its day and subsequently lost many of its supporters. We are reluctant to endorse any of them.

CASE REPORTS

Patient 5.1--Anisometropic Amblyopia

VISIT 1

Patient is a 15-year-old student. He has had glasses since age 6 but has used them only sporadically; in fact, he has not used them at all for the past six years. He consistently fails school vision-screening tests because of the poor visual acuity of his left eye. The youngster, himself, never voices complaints about his eyes. His school performance has always been average.

Chief Complaints

Patient has become interested in the possibility of obtaining an appointment to the United States Air Force Academy and has discovered that he is not likely to meet their physical standards because of inadequate visual acuity in his one eye. He has been informed that they require a corrected acuity of 20/20, each eye—with lenses, if necessary.

Salient Clinical Data

Health status: No evidence of pathology

Visual acuity (unaided): (OD) 20/20; (OS) 20/80

(*with old prescription*): (OD) 20/20; (OS) 20/60

Old prescription: (OD) +0.50 −0.25 cx 180
(OS) +2.00 −3.00 cx 165

Refractive status: Significant astigmatism, OS. Old lens prescription only partially compensates.

Lens prescription derived from today's examination:

(OD) +0.75 −0.50 cx 180 20/20
(OS) +4.00 −5.50 cx 165 20/60+

Binocular status (assessed through new lenses)

AT FAR
Orthophoria
Stereoacuity: 3 min of arc
Vergence facility: Unreliable measures; patient suppresses OS when prism is introduced.
Accommodation facility: Unreliable measures

AT NEAR
6 PD exophoria
Stereoacuity: 400 sec of arc

Vergence facility: Unreliable measures; patient suppresses OS when prism is introduced.
Accommodation facility: Unreliable measures

All else within normal limits.

Conclusion

Refractive amblyopia, OS. Patient's reduced visual acuity derives from marked anisometropia.

Prescription

Patient advised that his problem is not progressive; his visual acuity will not deteriorate further from this condition. In respect to his major concern, prognosis is not very favorable. Patient advised that remedial treatment may be instituted but that the prospect for acquiring 20/20 acuity from his left eye is very doubtful. Patient elects to attempt vision therapy anyhow; we agree on the basis that we will assess the effects of the therapy on a regular basis and terminate treatment when it becomes evident that further effort would not be worthwhile. Patient is to acquire new glasses (full presciption, as shown above) and wear them constantly for a week or two before vision therapy begins.

VISIT 2 (THREE WEEKS LATER)

Patient reports that he has worn new glasses fairly constantly for the past ten days. Initially, they caused him some discomfort and disorientation, but he now feels reasonably comfortable with them. Left eye visual acuity with glasses today is 20/50. No change in stereoacuity. Procedures 28 and 32 are dispensed along with the necessary equipment: a variable-mirror stereoscope and some cheiroscopic tracing patterns (simple line drawings that are supplied by the manufacturer of the stereoscope) for procedure 28; a red pencil and compatible red-green filters for procedure 32. Patient is asked to make a follow-up appointment for about three weeks hence.

VISIT 3 (THREE WEEKS LATER)

Patient reports compliance. He believes that he is seeing a little better with his left eye—at least, that is his impression when he engages in his training activities at home. Our assessment confirms this.

Left eye visual acuity: 20/40; OD unchanged (20/20)
Stereoacuity: At distance, 3 min of arc; at near, 100 sec of arc

Patient is informed of his progress in a way that does not lead him to believe that his goal—20/20—is at hand and advised to continue with his regimen unchanged.

VISIT 4 (THREE WEEKS LATER)

Patient reports continued compliance and, he believes, additional improvement in left eye visual acuity. Our assessment agrees: Left eye visual acuity, 20/40 +2.

Stereoacuity: At distance, 2 min of arc; at near, 80 sec of arc

Patient is informed that though he has progressed, he remains well away from his goal. Nonetheless, there has been improvement and further effort is probably justified.

Patient is advised to continue with same two procedures and add another, procedure 24. This latest one is designed to foster improved vergence and accommodation facility. In this case, that is not the primary objective; rather, it is a way of engaging the patient in an activity that will stimulate his awareness of stereopsis under different types of (accommodation and vergence) demand conditions. Patient is provided with the nonvariable-disparity tranaglyph and the red-green filters that the procedure calls for.

VISIT 5 (THREE WEEKS LATER)

Patient reports continued compliance but is not as optimistic about his progress; he does not think that his visual acuity has improved since last visit. Our assessment confirms his observations: left eye visual acuity is 20/40+. Stereoacuity at distance and near are the same as last visit.

Patient is advised accordingly and given the option of continuing or terminating treatment. We suggest (without being encouraging) that another month of effort might be worthwhile—but, then again, it might not. Patient elects to continue. No changes made in treatment.

VISIT 6 (THREE WEEKS LATER)

Patient reports compliance, but the erosion of his enthusiasm is evident. Our assessment shows no change in visual acuity or stereoacuity.

Patient is advised accordingly and assured that his efforts, albeit unsuccessful, were worthwhile and that he would be notified if some new and remarkable treatment method is reported in the future.

Case concluded.

Patient 5.2 Strabismus Amblyopia

VISIT 1

Patient is a 10-month-old male. His mother reports that his right eye has been crossed since birth and that the pediatrician suggested this visit when it became apparent that the child was not going to "grow out of it." No other pertinent facts revealed in history.

Salient Clinical Data

Health status: No evidence of pathology

Visual acuity: Preferential Looking procedure was unsuccessful; child did not respond to test conditions with sufficient reliability. It was established, however, that child was able to perceive (OU) a 2 mm candy bead from a distance of 0.5 m, suggesting a Snellen equivalent visual acuity of approximately 20/300. Patient objected vigorously to occlusion of his left eye; he was not nearly so energetic in reactions to occlusion of right eye, thereby indicating that right eye acuity is significantly lower than left eye acuity. Unable to take more precise measures.

Refractive status (with 1% Cyclogyl): (OD) +2.75 −1.50 cx 180; (OS) +2.00 −0.75 cx 180

Binocular status

AT FAR 40 PD constant right esotropia
Stereoacuity: Not measurable
Versions: Right eye restricted on right gaze; left eye shows no restrictions of movement.

AT NEAR 40 PD constant right esotropia. When retested through +3.50 D spheres (OU), continues to manifest 40 PD right esotropia.
Stereoacuity: Not measurable
Versions: Same as at distance; dextroversions of right eye are significantly restricted.

Conclusion

Infantile (congenital) esotropia; in addition, right eye is probably amblyopic, although this judgment was made on the basis of inference, not actual measures. Parent is informed that treatment should commence at once, with the initial concern being the apparent right eye amblyopia. Parent is further informed that treatment—patching—will not cure (eliminate) the strabismus; if successful, it will simply foster better visual acuity. The long-term prognosis for the strabismus is not favorable, except to the extent that surgery might improve the child's cosmetic appearance and, perhaps, facilitate the development of some peripheral fusion. (See chapter 6 for additional discussion.)

Prescription

A 2/1 patching regimen is instituted (see Table 5.1) and parent is asked to return with the child in about a week.

VISIT 2 (ONE WEEK LATER)

Parent reports compliance. Child has had constant occlusion since last visit: two days over left (good) eye, then one day over right eye, then two days over left eye, and so on.

Assessment indicates child now executes some dextroversions with his right eye. No other relevant changes observed.

Parent advised to continue with treatment and return in two weeks.

VISIT 3 (TWO WEEKS LATER)

Parent reports continued compliance.

Our assessment indicates further improvement. Child executes full dextroversions with his right eye. No other relevant changes observed.

Parent advised to continue with treatment.

VISIT 4 (TWO WEEKS LATER)

Parent again reports compliance.

Assessment reveals that the child now manifests sporadic episodes of alternating strabismus; there are occasions (with the patch removed) when his right eye will take up fixation and his left eye will assume the esotropic posture. In addition, the child is not quite so resistant to temporary occlusion of his left eye.

Refraction reveals no change from first visit. Lenses have never been prescribed. Consideration is given to that action now, with the inclusion of compensatory prisms to stimulate whatever binocular potential exists. Subsequent discussion ultimately leads to the conclusion that lenses that compensate for the refractive condition should be prescribed, with Fresnel prisms being added later, after the patching regimen has been stopped. We also advised the parent that unless significant positive changes are observed within the next few months, a surgical consultation would be appropriate.

VISIT 5 (ONE MONTH LATER)

Parent has continued patching regimen. Glasses have been procured and are worn without complaint. Child now manifests alternating strabismus and unrestricted motilities but still no signs of binocular potential or evidence that there is an innervational component contributing to the strabismus (see chapter 6, pp. 60–63).

Parent is advised to reduce patching to three hours per day over child's right eye. During the remainder of his waking hours, he is to be allowed to see with both eyes.

Compensatory prisms are attached to child's lenses (20 PD base out each lens) in an attempt to foster improved binocular function. Parent is advised that the prisms are not a cure; rather, they are an attempt to keep both eyes working simultaneously.

Next visit is scheduled for one week hence in order to monitor the effects of the prisms.

VISIT 6 (ONE WEEK LATER)

Parent has complied with new patching regimen. He reports that child wears his glasses without complaint. He also indicates that despite forewarnings he is disappointed because the child's eyes are still crossed.

Our assessment corroborates this observation. Child wears his glasses with apparent comfort; prisms continue to neutralize the deviation completely. Hence, parent is asked to continue with treatment but also is advised to obtain a surgical consultation whenever it is convenient. We suggest a specific ophthalmologist. Parent agrees.

VISIT 7 (ONE MONTH LATER)

Child was seen by the consulting surgeon a week ago. (We have already received a report.) His diagnosis confirms infantile (congenital) esotropia. His recommendation is for continuation of part-time patching and prisms for another few months, with re-assessment of refractive status regularly, keeping alert for any indications of an innervational component that might be contributing to the strabismus (see chapter 6). Given no change in the case findings, strabismus surgery is advised when the child is about 16 months old.

VISIT 8–10 (VISIT 10 THREE MONTHS AFTER VISIT 7)

Parent has complied. No changes have been observed in child's refractive status nor has any evidence of an innervational factor been documented.

Parent is referred back to surgeon; surgery is scheduled.

VISIT 11 (TWO MONTHS LATER)

Surgical procedure was carried out about one month ago with apparent (cosmetic) success. Child now manifests about 10 PD alternating esotropia. He rarely wears his glasses and seems to be visually comfortable. Parent is "delighted."

VISIT 14 (THREE YEARS LATER)

Child has been seen more or less annually since visit 11.

He is now about 4½ years old. He manifests a constant comitant right esotropia of about 10 PD diopters. He displays no restriction in ocular motilities. His refractive status is about the same in both eyes: +0.75 −0.25 cx 180. His unaided visual acuity is (OD) 20/25; (OS) 20/20. Stereoacuity is 3 min of arc at distance; 140 sec of arc at near. In brief, he has a small-angle strabismus with binocular function limited to peripheral fusion, but only a trivial right eye amblyopia (see pp. 57–58 for additional discussion regarding small-angle strabismus).

Child's condition is explained to parents as "much improved but not perfect." It should create no significant problems in his daily life, although it may limit his career choices slightly; for example, he probably would not be able to qualify for a position as a commercial airline pilot or some other activity that required precise stereoacuity. Parents are also forewarned that a good vision screening will detect the child's condition; he will fail the screening. Should this occur, they are simply to forward any forms to us. So long as we continue to see the child regularly, we will have no reservations about documenting his condition for the vision screener.

Parents are very pleased with outcomes; in fact, considering the nature of the case, so are we.

CHAPTER 6

Constant Strabismus

Patients with constant strabismus present considerable challenge. Some respond remarkably well to vision therapy; some, not at all. This chapter describes a systematic method for the primary-care optometrist to use in determining what treatment to recommend for different types of constant strabismus—which patients to reassure, which to refer for surgical consultation, which to provide with compensatory treatment, and which to provide with vision therapy. This last group is organized into two subgroups: those who usually can be satisfactorily treated in a primary-care practice and those who need the more comprehensive services of an optometrist specializing in strabismus therapy. The balance of the chapter is devoted to the clinical management of those patients who can be treated satisfactorily in a primary-care practice. Treatment of the other subgroup—those who should be referred to specialty practices—is not discussed; that topic goes beyond the scope of this book, and, indeed, there are already several excellent books available on the subject (see Bibliography).

IDENTIFICATION

Signs and Symptoms

Not all of the following are necessarily displayed or experienced by all patients.

1. Misalignment of one eye when the other eye fixates upon a given point in space.
2. Diplopia—Usually manifests only in patients who acquired strabismus well

past early childhood as the result of trauma, CNS lesion, and so forth, but may also be reported by individuals who engaged in extensive anti-suppression therapy that did not ultimately lead to a normal binocular status.

3. Head tilt or other unusual head posture—When this occurs in combination with strabismus, it is usually attributable to an extraocular muscle involvement or the nerve that innervates it.

Prevalence

Manifests in approximately 3 to 4 percent of the population.

Screening Tests

The tests listed below are organized into two clusters. The first will aid in detecting constant strabismus. The tests in the second cluster go beyond the detection process. They enable the optometrist to describe the condition in a way that will facilitate subsequent decisions about prognosis and treatment.

To Detect Constant Strabismus

1. *Unilateral cover test* at distance and near
2. *Hirschberg test.* This test is not nearly as sensitive or accurate as the cover test, but it is useful with very young patients who do not fixate on a target long enough for the practitioner to take valid cover test measures.
3. *Visual acuity, stereoacuity, and a test for central suppression* These three are listed together because in combination they comprise a test battery that is useful in identifying *microstrabismus,* a misalignment of the visual axes so slight that it is often very difficult to detect with the cover test—especially when you do not yet know that the patient is strabismic. In such cases, detection typically depends upon a process of inference that is based upon the presence of three clinical signs which, when they occur together, are usually referred to as the *monofixation syndrome:*

Reduced stereoacuity Worse than 100 sec of arc at distance; worse than 60 sec of arc at near.

Reduced (best-corrected) visual acuity in one eye Typically between 20/25 and 20/40, although it may be worse than 20/40.

Small central facultative scotoma (suppression area) in the deviating eye, which may be documented with the Worth Dot Test administered at near, mid-distance, and far, or with the 4 PD base-out test, or with various vectographic targets that are sensitive to suppression.

The first of these is conducted by starting off with the Worth Dot Test–apparatus held about 30 cm from the patient's eyes. Because of the proximity of the target, a fairly large area of each retina is stimulated. Hence, if the deviation (and suppression zone) is slight (e.g., less than 6 PD), suppression will not be detected. The patient will report seeing four dots. Then the apparatus is moved away from the patient. If there is a suppression zone in one eye, it will become evident because as the target distance increases a diminishing area of each retina is being stimulated by the lights of the Worth Dot Test apparatus. When the retinal area being stimulated becomes small enough to fall within the suppression zone, it will be revealed by the patient's reporting either two dots or three dots, depending upon which eye has the suppression zone and placement of the red-green filters.

The 4 PD base-out test is also designed to reveal a small suppression zone in one eye as follows: Patient fixates on a small far-point target (e.g., a single letter). Examiner holds a 4 D prism, base out, before one of the patient's eyes, watching the patient's eyes as he does this. If the eye behind the prism shifts toward the apex of the prism, it indicates that the eye perceived a shift in the location of the far-point target produced by the prism. This rules out a small suppression area in that eye unless, of course, the suppression area is smaller than 2 degrees—the magnitude of the shift of the target on retina that the 4 D prism produces. If the other eye, the one not behind the prism, is also observed to shift, it simply confirms Hering's law; but if the eye without the prism does not then make a fusional (recovery) movement, it suggests that this eye did not perceive diplopia. The inference is that there is a suppression zone in that eye. These observations can then be validated by placing the prism before the opposite eye and repeating the steps described above.*

To Describe Constant Strabismus. The following tests should be conducted with the patient wearing whatever lenses he needs to compensate fully for existing ametropia.

1. *Direction and magnitude* of the deviation at distance and near. These may be determined by:

   Unilateral cover test in combination with prisms. Take note of the amount and orientation of prism needed to reduce movement of the deviating eye to zero while the patient fixates at distance. Record the magnitude and direction of the deviation. Repeat at near fixation. Make certain that the patient is truly fixating on the target and keeping it clear. When measuring at near point, it often helps to shift the target a bit—to the left and right—as you conduct this test, watching the patient's eyes as you do this. A difference of more than 10 PD between distance and near fixation in the direction of less exotropia or more esotropia at near suggests that innervational factors are contributing to the strabismus. Interpret this to be a *favorable sign* (the relevance of this is discussed below). Repeat with opposite eye fixating. If a difference in magnitude is observed, consider the strabismus to be noncomitant.

   Hirschberg test As acknowledged above, this test is acceptable only when the patient does not maintain fixation long enough for a cover test to be conducted (i.e., with very young children). Hence, it is useful for near-point measures only. Record the difference between the two corneal reflections in 0.5-mm increments.

*The patient referred to in chapter 4 (see p. 28) who appears to manifest intermittent strabismus but is not able to demonstrate good stereoacuity—even when his eyes "look straight"—is probably best thought of as a constant strabismic with two anomalous binocular states: one, a readily apparent, large-angle strabismus; the other, an unapparent, microstrabismus. Such patients often exhibit the monofixation syndrome when in the latter posture.

Transform this into prism diopters (1 mm difference = approximately 22 PD of deviation).

2. *Comitance* When the magnitude of deviation remains constant in all directions of gaze, it is called *comitant*. When the deviation varies more than 10 PD as a function of the direction of gaze, it is called *incomitant* or *noncomitant*. Comitance may be determined by the cover test or Hirschberg test conducted as the patient fixates in different directions. Also look for a difference between primary and secondary deviation (i.e., difference in the magnitude of deviation that depends upon which eye is fixating). If noncomitance is observed, take note of the relative differences in the deviation as a function of the position of gaze. There is no need for exact measures at this time. Knowing the precise amount of noncomitance does not affect the optometrist's decision regarding when or how to proceed with vision therapy, although it might eventually influence his or her decision regarding the relative merits of reassurance, surgery, or compensatory lenses as appropriate treatment in those cases where vision therapy is not recommended.

3. *Frequency* This may be determined by direct observation, case history, and stereoacuity tests. If there is valid evidence that the patient is able to achieve a normal binocular status (as defined in chapter 4) at any time, then the diagnosis of constant strabismus is wrong. Hence, the information in this chapter does not pertain; the patient displays intermittent strabismus, and chapter 4 should be consulted instead (see the discussion in chapter 4, p. 28, regarding differentiating between constant and intermittent strabismus).

4. *Laterality* May be determined by direct observation and comparison of right and left eye visual acuities. The patient with 20/20 acuity in each eye is not apt to have a unilateral strabismus; if he did, it would probably be reflected in a lowered acuity in the deviating eye. Similarly, the patient with 20/20 in one eye and 20/200 in the other is not likely to have an alternating strabismus. For all practical purposes, this factor is important primarily because of how it relates to amblyopia.

5. *Visual acuity* This information is used to identify or rule out unilateral amblyopia. If significant amblyopia exists (best corrected visual acuity is 20/50 or worse), it should be addressed *before* any major effort is made to stimulate normal binocular function.

6. *The effect of extra plus or minus spheres* Here, again, innervational factors are the focus of attention. Binocular misalignment is reduced in some constant strabismus patients with plus or minus lenses that go beyond what is called for by their ametropia (i.e., lenses that relax or stimulate accommodation). It therefore is useful to investigate this possibility empirically by placing minus or plus lenses before the strabismic patient's eyes and measuring their effect on the deviation. For example, if patient is an exotrope, assess the effect of about −2.50 to −4.00 D spheres (OU) as the patient fixates on a near and then a distant target. If patient is an esotrope, assess the effect of about +2.50 to +4.00 D spheres (OU) as the patient fixates on a near target.

Consider any reduction in deviation in excess of 10 PD to be a *favorable sign*. How this information is to be used will be discussed shortly.

7. *Patient's potential for normal fusion and stereopsis* It has already been

established that the patient lacks central fusion. That is one of the characteristics that earned him the diagnosis of constant strabismus in the first place. It is not yet established, however, whether the patient is capable of fusion when appropriate targets have been positioned so that both maculae are stimulated simultaneously, despite their misalignment (i.e., through use of compensatory prisms).

Determine whether the patient is capable of such fusion in the following manner:

a. Place sufficient prism in front of the patient's eyes to neutralize the strabismus at distance and administer the Worth Dot Test at 6 m in moderate illumination. Then remove the prism and repeat the test.

If the patient reports seeing two, three, or five dots (i.e., suppression or diplopia) when the prism is not in place and four dots (fusion) when the prism is in place, interpret it as a *favorable sign*. It is evidence of potential for normal fusion (second-degree, at the least); this will influence your prognosis (see below).

If the patient reports four dots under both conditions, and if he truly is a constant strabismic, it suggests that the patient is unreliable; hence, the data derived from this test are of no use.

If the patient reports seeing four dots without the prism and something different than that when the prism is in place, it suggests *anomalous retinal correspondence* (ARC) (see below).

If the patient reports seeing two, three, or five dots both when the prism is and is not in place, it raises doubts about his potential for normal fusion.

b. Assess the patient's ability to perceive stereopsis at near, without the prism (e.g., using the Titmus Stereotest Fly, or test card 9 from the Keystone Basic Binocular Test). Obviously, stereoacuity—if it is elicited at all—will be poor; the patient is strabismic, after all. Then repeat the test through the prism. If the prism improves the patient's stereoacuity, interpret it as a *favorable sign*. It is evidence of potential for normal stereopsis.

TREATMENT

Factors the Optometrist Should Consider

Prognosis for Remediation Through Vision Therapy. The procedures described above mark the end of the initial testing. It is now time to make some interim, or perhaps final, decisions about the feasibility of remediation through vision therapy. The critical factors in making this determination are the extent to which the strabismus can be linked to innervational factors, and the patient's potential for fusion and stereopsis.

Four tests were described above in which favorable signs might or might not be observed. In reverse order of presentation (as shown in Figure 6.1), but in correct order in terms of relative importance, they were (1) the effect of compensating prisms on the patient's stereoacuity; (2) the effect of compensating prisms on the patient's fusional ability (Worth Dot Test); (3) the effect of fixation distance (far and near) on the magnitude of the deviation; and (4) the effect of plus or minus spheres on the magnitude of the deviation. The first two of these—and to some extent the latter

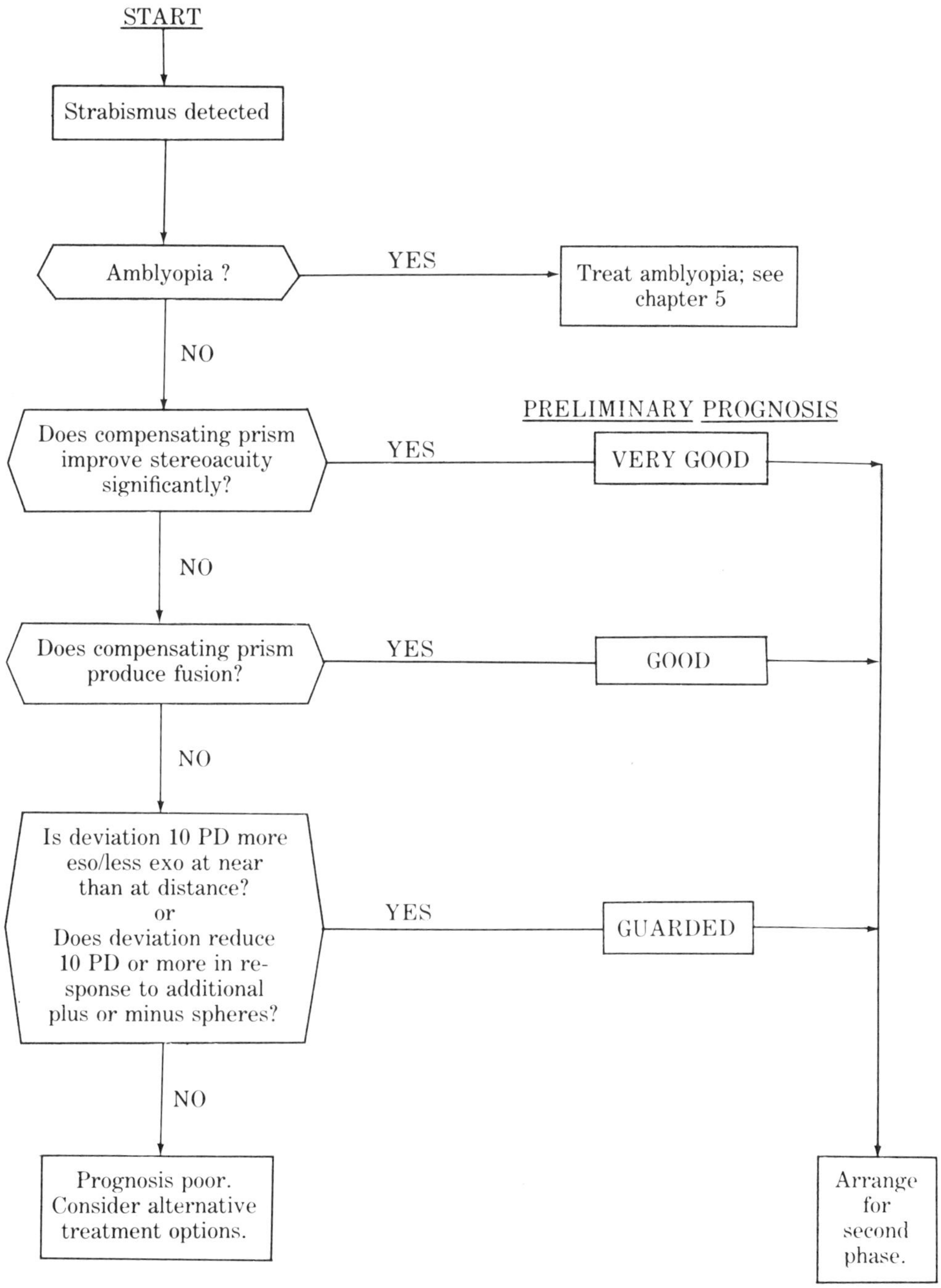

FIGURE 6.1 Diagnostic Sequence for Constant Strabismus: First Phase

two as well—presume that the patient manifests good visual acuity in both eyes (i.e., at least 20/40). If he does not, then the diagnostic validity of these procedures is significantly reduced. Hence, as shown in Figure 6.1, the amblyopia should be addressed first.

If the first of these tests (the effect of compensating prism on stereopsis) yields a *favorable sign*, the patient should be viewed, at least thus far, as a very good candidate for vision therapy.

If compensating prism does not improve stereoacuity, but does enable the patient to display normal fusion (i.e., with the Worth Dot Test), then, again, he probably is a good candidate for vision therapy, but not quite so good as if he responds positively to the stereoacuity stimuli.

If the patient does not respond favorably in either of these two situations, but does display a significant reduction in the angle of deviation when accommodation is stimulated or inhibited (by changing fixation distance or by introducing minus or plus lenses), then prognosis, although certainly more guarded, is not completely negative. In any of the above situations, a second visit for additional diagnostic testing is warranted.

On the other hand, if none of the above procedures yields a *favorable sign*, then the prognosis for remediation through vision therapy is very poor. For all practical purposes, there is no good reason for a second visit.

Alternative Treatment Options. The optometrist should discuss these with the patient at the end of the first or second visit, depending upon the decision process outlined above.

Reassurance This treatment is appropriate for those patients who show no potential for normal binocular fusion or stereopsis as defined above and whose strabismus is not cosmetically objectionable.

Referral Assuming that pathology has been ruled out, referral to an optometric colleague who has developed special skills and knowledge in the treatment of strabismus with vision therapy may be justified. A poor prognosis does not necessarily mean an impossible situation; however, such a referral should always include qualifying statements to the patient that speak honestly to the prognosis. Surgical consultation is appropriate for those patients whose constant strabismus is cosmetically objectionable and who do not display the intellectual, motivational, or physiological characteristics—including any potential for normal binocular function—that would warrant further consideration of vision therapy.

Compensation This treatment is appropriate in three situations: (1) for those patients who do display the potential for normal binocular vision but lack the intellectual or motivational traits needed to benefit from vision therapy; (2) for those patients who experience constant diplopia that is not attributable to an active pathology, and which can be substantially reduced, or perhaps even eliminated, by accurate application of compensatory prism (e.g., muscle paresis); and (3) for those few patients whose cosmetic appearance improves when base-in or base-out prism is held before one or both of their eyes. This latter treatment does not affect binocular function at all; it simply alters the patient's appearance in a way that is desirable in some cases.

If Patient Accepts Recommendation for Second Visit

When dealing with constant strabismus, a secure decision regarding the advisability for, and design of, a vision therapy program usually requires more testing than is described above; that is, a second visit to examine more extensively those patients who displayed *favorable signs*—whose strabismus appears to be linked, at least in part, to innervational factors and who demonstrate potential for normal binocular fusion and, perhaps, stereopsis. Hence, the recommendation offered at the end of the first visit in such cases is that vision therapy may be recommended but, then again, it may not. Such a decision is more easily made at the end of the second visit. Obviously, the enthusiasm with which this is said depends upon the number of favorable signs observed during the above-described assessment.

On the basis of the knowledge obtained during the first visit, the following test should be carried out at the second visit (see also Figure 6.2):

VECTOTRAINER

(See procedure 25 in Procedures Manual.)

1. Insert a pair of quoit vectograms into the vectotrainer set at the position that should compensate for the patient's strabismus at near. (This information is available from your measurement of the magnitude of his deviation; see p. 58.) Patient wears Polaroid filters.

2. Measure patient's objective angle of deviation under these conditions. Occlude one of patient's eyes and have him fixate, with the other eye, on one specific location on the quoit (e.g., the circle that contains the suppression *control mark*). Now move the occluder to the other eye and, again, have him fixate on the same place on that quoit. Watch his eyes as you move the occluder from one eye to the other. If you observe eye movements (i.e., refixating), change the relative positions of the two vectograms so as to neutralize them. When the occluder no longer elicits eye movements, take note of and record the setting of the vectograms. This represents the *objective angle of deviation* under these conditions. It should agree with what you initially measured. If it does not, then recheck your measurements, making sure that the patient is exercising adequate accommodation as you do this (i.e., keeping the fixation target clear).

3. The patient (with both eyes fixating) should report seeing a single (fused) target. If he does, go to step 4. If he does not see a single target, have him re-adjust the positions of the vectograms so that the targets are fused. If only a small re-adjustment is needed, go to the next step. On the other hand, if the patient repositions the vectograms so that they are at, or close to, zero (or anywhere else that differs significantly from his objective angle) instead of where his angle of deviation would predict—thereby demonstrating ARC—stop this procedure and go to the next, Variable-Mirror Stereoscope.

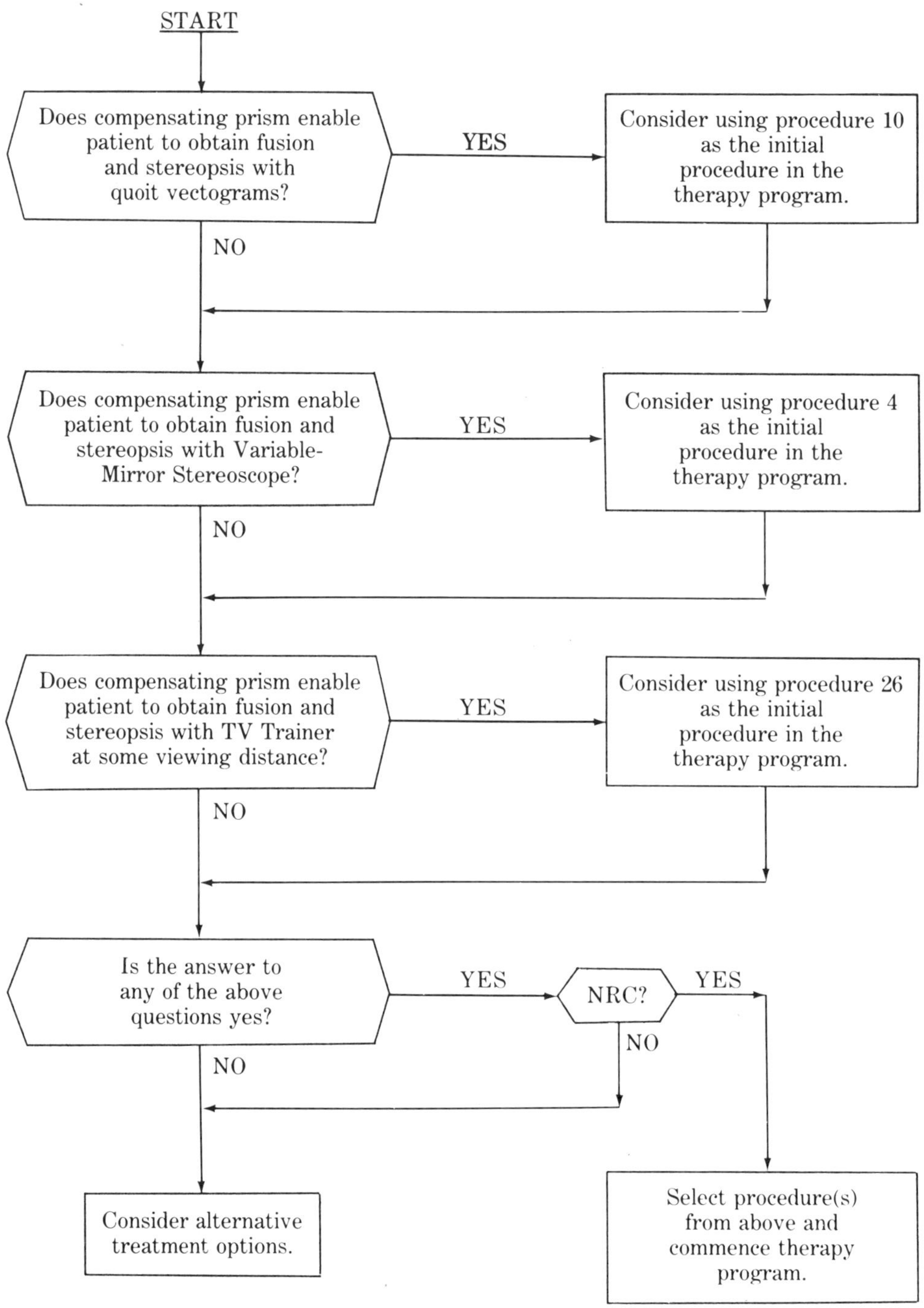

FIGURE 6.2 Diagnostic Sequence for Constant Strabismus: Second Phase

4. Have the patient change the relative positions of the vectograms a small amount, first in one direction, then in the other (e.g., 2 to 4 PD), and ask him to describe what he sees as he is doing this.

5. *Optimal response:* Patient reports an illusion of stereopsis that changes in accord with his shifting of the vectograms; the fused quoit appears to move closer (and become smaller) and farther away (and become larger) in synchrony with the relative positions of the vectograms. If this occurs, go on to step 7 below; if not, go to step 6.*

6. If the patient does not give the *optimal response*—if he does not obtain the illusion of change in size or relative position of the target—stop this procedure and go on to the next, Variable-Mirror Stereoscope.

7. If the patient does give the *optimal response*, measure his vergence ranges with the vectotrainer; that is, determine the limits of his ability to maintain fusion and stereopsis as the prism demand is changed in both directions. Record this and go on to the next procedure.

VARIABLE-MIRROR STEREOSCOPE

(*See procedure 27 in Procedures Manual.*)

1. Insert a pair of third-degree fusion targets (targets containing stereopsis stimuli; e.g., eccentric circles) into the side panels of the Variable-Mirror Stereoscope and position the mirrors at the location that should compensate for the strabismus. (This data should be available from your measurement of the magnitude of his near-point deviation; see p. 58.)

2. Measure patient's objective angle of deviation under these conditions. Occlude one of patient's eyes and have him fixate with the other eye at one specific location on the target. Now move the occluder to the other eye and have him fixate again at the same location on that target. Watch his eyes as you move the occluder from one eye to the other. If you observe eye movements (i.e., refixating), change the relative position of the mirrors so as to neutralize them. When the occluder no longer elicits eye movements, take note of and record the setting of the mirrors. This represents the objective angle under these conditions.

3. The patient should report seeing a single (fused) target that has the illusion of depth (three-dimensionality). If he does, go to step 4. If he does not see a single stereoscopic target, have him re-adjust the positions of the mirrors so

* The distance and size change illusions are produced by the relative positions of the two vectograms. When the patient is looking through the filters, each vectogram can be seen by one eye only. If the vectograms are placed in *crossed disparity*—that is, so that the vectogram visible to the patient's right eye is to the left of the vectogram that is visible to the patient's left eye—the patient will have to converge in order to fuse them, and the fused target will appear to be closer and smaller. If the opposite condition is presented—*uncrossed disparity*, where the vectogram visible to the patient's right eye is to the right of the vectogram that is visible to the patient's left eye—the patient will have to diverge in order to fuse them, and the fused target will appear to be larger and farther away. Hence, if there is some question about the validity or reliability of the patient's responses, it may be tested by re-orienting the vectograms or the Polaroid filters so that they are upside down. This will reverse the apparent location of the fused target; that is, if the quoit originally appeared to be floating in front of the vectogram holder, it will now appear to be floating behind the holder and have become larger, and vice versa. See pp. 131–133 for more discussion regarding this topic.

that the targets are fused. If only a small re-adjustment is needed, go on to step 4. On the other hand, if the patient repositions the mirrors so that they are at, or close to, zero (or anywhere else that differs significantly from his objective angle) instead of where his angle of deviation would predict—thereby demonstrating ARC—stop this procedure and go on to the next, TV Trainer.

4. Have the patient change the relative positions of the mirrors a small amount, first in one direction, then in the other (e.g., 2 to 4 PD) and ask him to describe what he sees as he is doing this. (Moving the mirrors closer together requires the eyes to converge in order to continue to fuse the two images; moving the mirrors apart requires the eyes to diverge in order to maintain fusion.)

5. *Optimal response* Patient reports that the illusion of stereopsis remains. If this occurs, go on to step 8, below; if not, go to step 6. (Patient may also report that the size of the target changes in accord with his shifting of the mirrors, appearing to become somewhat smaller or larger, but because these changes are not great, they may not be noticed.)

6. If the patient does not give the optimal response, replace the third-degree (stereo) targets with second-degree (flat-fusion) targets and repeat steps 1 through 4, above. For the *optimal response* now, the patient reports fusion but no illusion of depth.

7. If the patient does not give an optimal response as defined in steps 5 or 6, stop this procedure and go on to the next, TV Trainer.

8. If the patient gives the optimal response to either the third- or second-degree targets, test his vergence ranges with the mirror stereoscope and those targets; that is, measure the limits of his ability to maintain fusion and stereopsis as the prism demand is changed in both directions. Record this and go on to the next procedure.

ANAGLYPH TV TRAINER*

(See procedure 26 in Procedures Manual.)

1. Position the TV trainer in front of a television screen, or any other suitable visual stimulus that is larger than the TV Trainer itself and is visible to the patient from a 6-m distance.

2. Before placing the anaglyph spectacles on the patient, have him report what he sees. The only acceptable (i.e., possible) response is that he sees the entire stimulus—part of it through the red plastic, part through the green—and some red and green letters and circles at the edges of the plastic. If the patient does not report this, attempt to establish the source of confusion; do not go on until this has been resolved.

3. Position the patient about 6 m from the stimulus. Have him view it through the anaglyph spectacles and report what he sees.

4. If the patient reports seeing the entire stimulus, more or less the way it appeared before he put on the anaglyph spectacles, suspect one of two possibilities: (1) The original diagnosis was incorrect—he does not have constant strabismus;

* The Polaroid TV Trainer is a satisfactory substitute.

if he has strabismus at all, it is intermittent, thereby explaining his ability to respond to this situation in the way a person with normal binocular vision would. (2) Patient is manifesting ARC. Therefore, if the patient gives this response, re-assess the original diagnosis (see tests, above). If it is correct, assume ARC under these conditions, stop this procedure and move on to step 9.

5. If the patient reports that he sees only that portion of the screen that is visible to his fixating eye—that the other area is "blank"—place enough prism before the patient's eye(s) to compensate for his deviation (i.e., the objective angle) at 6 m and repeat step 3, above.

6. *Optimal response:* Patient reports seeing the entire stimulus, more or less the way it appeared before he put on the anaglyph spectacles with the exception that the pairs of circles along the side now present the illusion of depth.

7. If the patient does not give the optimal response—that is, if he reports that the neutralizing prism produced no change in what he sees—go on to step 9.

8. If the patient gives the optimal response, measure his fusional ranges under those conditions with a prism bar; that is, measure his ability to maintain fusion while increasing amounts of prism, base out and base in, are held before his eyes.

9. Regardless of response—optimal or not—repeat all the above TV Trainer tests (starting with step 1) at both 3 and 0.5 m distances.

Anomalous Retinal Correspondence. Many books and papers have been devoted to this topic, and no attempt is made here to summarize that information.* Rather, we suggest that the most profitable way for the primary-care practitioner to conceptualize ARC is to understand it operationally, as illustrated above. In effect, ARC describes a situation wherein the patient responds to a given set of conditions *as though* he had normal binocular vision, yet the examiner is able to observe a misalignment of the visual axes. The patient's subjective responses indicate that he has normal binocular vision; the optometrist's objective measures on this same occasion show that not to be the case.

The practical importance of identifying ARC is that one of the fundamental principles of vision therapy is to determine what the patient can do that is desirable and then to build on that (see pp. 1–2). The patient with ARC is deceptive. If his responses are taken literally, one can conclude that he performs normally under certain conditions (see Vectotrainer, Variable-Mirror Stereoscope, and TV Trainer, above). Hence, in theory, the vision therapy program could commence at that point, with the patient engaging in activities that build on his already established capacity to function binocularly under those conditions. In fact, however, his binocular vision is not normal; it is based on anomalous retinal correspondence. Vision therapy that builds upon that foundation is only enhancing an undesirable phenomenon. This does not imply that ARC is "bad." On the contrary, it is a reasonably good adaptation to a bad situation—strabismus. It enables the patient to use both his eyes simultaneously. What it does not do is give the patient the appearance of alignment or good stereoacuity.

To identify ARC There are many standardized tests for ARC. There is no

* See Bibliography for a representative selection.

practical purpose, however, in discussing them here. The methods described above will serve the primary-care optometrist very well; in fact, they are more useful than the standard tests because they examine the patient's retinal correspondence under the same conditions in which therapy will be done—if it is done. This is why we suggested, above, that the potential for binocular function be tested in three or four different situations; it is possible to show ARC under one set of conditions and NRC under another. Obviously, if a condition is discovered wherein the patient displays potential for binocular vision *and* normal retinal correspondence, that would be the place to start vision therapy.

Factors the Optometrist Should Consider at the End of the Second Visit

Prognosis for Remediation Through Vision Therapy. As illustrated in Figure 6.2, the critical factor in making this determination is the patient's potential for fusion and stereopsis under the test conditions described above.

If an optimal response to stereopsis targets was obtained in *any* of the tests prescribed above (Vectotrainer, Variable-Mirror Stereoscope, TV Trainer—at any test distance in the last of these), then prognosis for vision therapy is favorable. If such a response was obtained in *all* of the tests, then prognosis is very favorable.

If an optimal response was not obtained when stereopsis targets were used but was obtained from second-degree targets used in conjunction with the Variable-Mirror Stereoscope or TV Trainer procedures, then the prognosis is less optimistic, but not completely unfavorable.

In both of the above circumstances, vision therapy should be offered, but the patient should not be led to believe that success is guaranteed; only that some investment of time, energy, and money is worth making. In other words, do not "sell." Present the prospects to the patient in an encouraging but objective way and reserve the right to stop the vision therapy effort if progress does not occur as anticipated.

If an optimal response was not obtained in any of the procedures, then consider offering reassurance (if the strabismus is cosmetically acceptable), referral to a colleague who specializes in strabismus vision therapy, or referral for surgical consultation (see alternative treatment options, p. 62).

Factors the Patient Should Consider

Probable Outcome of Treatment. It is possible that the patient will ultimately achieve normal binocular alignment and that he will appreciate normal stereopsis; the better his entering level, the better his prospects. It is not wise or accurate, however, to make this statement in too enthusiastic a manner until after there has been time to assess what the beginning therapy efforts produce. A great deal of time and effort is usually needed to replace the undesirable habit of strabismus with the desirable habit of normal binocular vision.

It is generally advisable, therefore, to commence the treatment, encourage the patient to exert the necessary effort on a daily basis, reassess the patient regularly, about once every two weeks, and reconsider the prognosis and recommendation for vision therapy at monthly intervals.

Progress is rarely steady and even; there will probably be advances that occur in bursts, then periods of no change. If progress is made, however, it will be apparent at the monthly follow-up sessions—not necessarily by a gradually diminishing angle of deviation but, rather, by a gradually increasing ability to overcome the existing binocular condition. As the constant strabismic improves, he will learn how to maintain alignment, first with, then without, compensatory prisms. Eventually, if he continues to progress, he will become an intermittent strabismic; then, after additional effort and learning, he will display the characteristics of a binocular patient with vergence infacility. Eventually, he will become a normally functioning binocular individual (see additional comments in this regard in chapter 4, p. 31).

Consequences If Recommendations Are Not Followed. A lack of compliance will result in the continuation of present signs and symptoms. Except for the very young patient, there is little danger of the binocular status deteriorating further. With the young patient, there is a real risk of amblyopia or ARC (see additional comments on p. 73).

Patient's Obligations. The patient will be required to engage in about 30 to 45 minutes of prescribed remedial activities daily, perhaps for as long as one year; this to be followed by another 6 to 12 months of maintenance activities that require about 5 to 10 minutes per day.†

Number and Frequency of Office Visits. The following are rough estimates because there is no way of predicting the rate at which individual patients will progress. A better estimate is possible after the patient has engaged in vision therapy for a month or two. By that time, the optometrist is able to judge the patient's willingness to adhere to a daily regimen, his capacity to learn from the activities, and the effects of his efforts to date. On average, if the patient places in level I, successful treatment of constant strabismus requires from 15 to 30 office visits. If patient places in level II, approximately 10 to 15 fewer visits are needed.

Implementation of Vision Therapy

Steps to be taken once the patient elects to accept the recommendation for vision therapy:

1. Schedule Patient for the Next (Third) Visit. At that visit, the office assistant will explain and dispense activities that were selected on the basis of data collected at the second visit. In effect, the placement process occurred during the second visit.

2. Placement Testing. Levels and goals, organized in descending order of difficulty (see also Table 6.1).

† It is precarious to attempt to predict the time required for the successful treatment of constant strabismus. The projection of "perhaps for as long as one year" stated above is probably an overstatement in many cases; however, the projection of "another 6 to 12 months of maintenance activities" is not an overstatement. This phase of the treatment is essential to establishing the newly learned behaviors as habitual.

LEVEL III

There are two goals for this level. In both, the patient is to be able to demonstrate the respective behavior without the aid of compensatory prisms but with the aid of facilitating (plus or minus spherical) lenses if they are needed:

a. Patient is able to execute fusional vergence jumps as follows:

AT FAR	From 3 PD base in *to* plano, and vice versa*
	From 3 PD base out *to* plano, and vice versa*
AT NEAR	From 6 PD base in *to* plano, and vice versa*
	From 6 PD base out *to* plano, and vice versa*

b. Patient experiences and reports physiological diplopia immediately upon being presented with appropriate stimuli and the request to fixate on one of them (e.g., a row of letters at 20 ft and a penlight at 16 in).

LEVEL II

There are two goals for this level also. In both, as with level III, the patient is to be able to demonstrate the respective behaviors without the aid of compensatory prisms but with the aid of facilitating (plus or minus spherical) lenses, if they are needed.

a. Patient is able to maintain binocular alignment at distance *and* at near.
b. Patient is able to execute fusional vergence jumps as follows:

AT FAR	From 2 PD base in *to* plano, and vice versa*
	From 2 PD base out *to* plano, and vice versa,* *or*
AT NEAR	From 3 PD base in *to* plano, and vice versa*
	From 3 PD base out *to* plano, and vice versa*

LEVEL I

Patient is able to maintain binocular alignment at distance *or* at near, without the aid of compensatory prisms, but with the aid of facilitating (plus or minus spherical) lenses if they are needed.

Obviously, the final goal (level III) does not define a satisfactory completion to the treatment of constant strabismus. Rather, that goal represents the patient's transition from constant to intermittent strabismus. Once level III is achieved, therefore, the patient should be treated as an intermittent strabismic, in accord with the information presented in chapter 4. In fact, the level III goal for constant strabismus is identical to the level I goals in the intermittent strabismus and vergence infacility regimens.

---

* Sixty cycles within 5 minutes. For one cycle, start with fusion and clarity through base-in prism (loose, hand-held, or mounted in flippers); then fusion and clarity when prism is removed, then fusion and clarity again through base in. Repeat, base out–plano–base out. Test at far, then at near.

TABLE 6.1 Constant Strabismus Treatment Goals[a]

	Prism power (PD)				
	Far		Near		
Level	**Base in**	**Base out**	**Base in**	**Base out**	**Cycle[b]**
III	3	3	6	6	Plano to prism to plano
	Patient experiences physiological diplopia immediately upon being presented with appropriate conditions.				
II	2	2	3	3	Plano to prism to plano
I	Single, simultaneous, binocular vision at far *or* at near as demonstrated by fusion/stereopsis; i.e., evidence that strabismus has changed from constant to intermittent at one or more fixation distances.				

[a] Patient to demonstrate capabilities without the aid of compensating prisms, but with the aid of facilitating (plus or minus spherical) lenses if they are needed.
[b] Rate = 60 cycles within 5 minutes.

Patient's Performance. During visit 2, the patient demonstrated that he could obtain fusion and, perhaps, stereopsis *if* conditions were arranged that made it possible for his two macular areas to be stimulated simultaneously despite his strabismus, by using prisms that compensated for the strabismus or an instrument that allowed the targets to be positioned where desired. Also documented at that visit were the patient's vergence ranges under those conditions. That represents the patient's baseline level. His next efforts will be devoted to extending those ranges, as follows:

Prescribe appropriately compensating prisms for the patient for full-time wear (i.e., lenses that will cause both maculae to be stimulated simultaneously). Fresnel lenses are usually best because they can easily be replaced as the patient makes progress and requires less prism to obtain alignment; however, they do reduce visual acuity somewhat, and this may be a consideration in some cases.

Identify in Table 6.2 one of the procedures with which the patient demonstrated the optimal response (i.e., fusion and stereopsis with Vectotrainer, Variable-Mirror Stereoscope, or TV Trainer.)

Locate that procedure in the Procedures Manual, photocopy it, and amend those instructions in accord with the patient's needs. For example, say the patient obtained stereopsis with the Variable-Mirror Stereoscope mirrors set at 20 PD base out. You therefore add 10 D of base-out prism to each of the patient's lenses. Hence, the patient will begin his activities with the mirrors of the stereoscope set at zero. His goal is to extend his vergence ranges in both directions (see procedure 4). Then follow the general sequence described in chapter 1. Make certain to redetermine, regularly, the amount of prism the patient needs in order to obtain fusion. Even though we do not expect his deviation to reduce in magnitude at the onset, we do expect his ability to cope with that deviation to improve. As

TABLE 6.2 Constant Strabismus Procedures

Procedure	Apparatus	Targets	This procedure is appropriate if the patient is to start therapy at		Prerequisites[a]
			Far	Near	
4	Variable-Mirror Stereoscope; compensating prisms	Second- and third-degree targets positioned at the objective angle		X	A or C
10	Vectotrainer; polarizers; compensating prisms	Quoit vectograms positioned at ortho		X	A
25	Vectogram; polarizers	Quoit vectograms positioned at the objective angle		X	A
26	TV Trainer; red-green filters; compensating prisms	TV set at far, near, or anywhere between	X	X	A or B or C or D
27	Variable-Mirror Stereoscope	Second- and third-degree targets		X	A or C

[a] Prerequisites: A = third-degree fusion (i.e., stereopsis) at near when strabismus is neutralized by prisms or placement of targets; B = third-degree fusion at far when strabismus is neutralized by prisms and/or placement of targets; C = second-degree fusion (i.e., single, simultaneous, binocular vision) at near when strabismus is neutralized by prisms and/or placement of targets; D = second-degree fusion at far when strabismus is neutralized by prisms or placement of targets.

this occurs—as his fusional ranges increase—he should require less prism to accomplish the same status.

There is an alternative to using prisms. Have the patient begin his training activities with the instrument set at the position that enables him to obtain fusion. His goal in this approach is same: to increase fusional vergence ranges in both directions from that starting point (see, for example, procedure 27). This method may be preferred with some patients, depending upon their reaction to the cosmetic appearance and spatial distortions of the prism.

QUESTIONS AND ANSWERS ABOUT CONSTANT STRABISMUS

Q. How should the constant strabismic with amblyopia (best-corrected visual acuity is 20/50 or worse) be managed?

A. Address the amblyopia first (see chapter 5 and Figure 6.1). If amblyopia therapy is successful, then go on to the strabismus. If amblyopia therapy is not successful, the prognosis for treatment of strabismus with vision therapy is significantly less favorable.

Q. Vision therapy is not feasible for very young children with constant strabismus. How then should they be managed?

A. The following guidelines apply (see also the case report of patient 5.2 in chapter 5, pp. 52–55):

1. Make certain that the child is provided with whatever lenses he needs to compensate fully for existing ametropia.
2. Provide sufficient prism to compensate for the deviation; also provide whatever additional spherical lens power is called for to facilitate alignment; for example, plus spheres—at near only, of course—for the esotrope, and minus spheres—at near and distance or at distance only (depending upon the magnitude of the strabismus at those fixation distances)—for the exotrope. When prescribing prisms, it is often best to use Fresnel prisms or spheres first. If the patient does not adapt to them, if they continue to neutralize the deviation after a week or two of wear, have the prisms or spheres incorporated into the lens. If, instead, he does adapt, if his eyes return to a strabismic position despite the prisms, discard them.
3. Take whatever action is needed to reduce or prevent amblyopia (see chapter 5).
4. Re-assess the child's ametropia and binocular status on a regular basis, updating and expanding the treatment program when feasible.
5. If there is no evidence that the strabismus is, at least in part, linked with an innervational component—a situation more common among infantile (congenital) strabismics than those who do not manifest a deviation until after their first birthdays—then give serious consideration to recommending a referral for surgical consultation. Most pediatric ophthalmologists seem to agree that the optimum time for surgery for congenital strabismus is when the baby is about 12 to 18 months old. It should also be pointed out that successful surgery in those cases does not imply normal binocular vision; typically, it means that the patient will have the appearance of "straight eyes" and, in some cases, be able to display some gross (peripheral) stereopsis.

CASE REPORTS

Patient 6.1—Esotropia (Favorable Prognosis)

VISIT 1

Patient is a 12-year-old male.

Chief Complaints: Patient has a long history of esotropia. Condition was first noted in left eye when child was about 19 months old. First glasses and patching therapy was prescribed when he was 2 years old. Patching was discontinued after about three months, at which time patient underwent strabismus surgery. According to his parents, the operation helped, but he still looked a little "cross-eyed," even when he wore his glasses. Parents are now concerned about child's cosmetic appearance and are very interested in vision therapy as a means of "straightening his eyes" and eliminating glasses. Early photographs of the child, taken before his strabismus surgery, indicate a significant left esotropia; approximately 40 to 50 PD.

Salient Clinical Data

Health status: No evidence of pathology

Visual acuity (old prescription): (OD) 20/20; (OS) 20/30+

Refractive status: (OU) +5.00 −0.75 cx 90 (no change from old prescription)

Binocular status (with prescription)

Cover test

AT FAR	10 PD constant, comitant, alternating esotropia (OD is preferred eye.)
AT NEAR	25 PD constant, comitant, alternating esotropia (OD is preferred eye.)

Measured through additional +2.50 D spheres (OU): 10 PD constant esotropia

Worth Dot Test (with prescription)

AT FAR	Alternating suppression (OD is preferred eye.)
AT NEAR	Alternating suppression (OD is preferred eye.)

Worth Dot Test (with prescription, compensating prisms, and, at near, additional +2.50-D spheres)

AT FAR	Fusion
AT NEAR	Fusion

Stereoacuity (with prescription):

AT FAR	4 min of arc (AO vectographic slide)
AT NEAR	400 sec of arc (Titmus animals)

Stereoacuity (with prescription, compensating prisms, and, at near, additional +2.50-D spheres)

AT FAR	3 min of arc (AO vectographic slide)
AT NEAR	100 sec of arc (Titmus stereotest)

The above data enable us to determine a preliminary prognosis as follows (see pp. 58–62 and Figure 6.1):

Effect of fixation distance: Esotropia increases significantly when fixation is shifted from distance to near. This is a *favorable sign.*

Effect of additional +2.50 D spheres (OU) at near: Deviation markedly reduced. This is a *favorable sign* (see p. 59).

Effect of compensating prisms on Worth Dot Test: Stable fusion. This is a *favorable sign* (see p. 60).

Effect of compensating prisms on stereopsis

AT FAR — Stereoacuity improves from 4 min of arc to 3 min of arc; however, this could also be attributed to monocular cues.

AT NEAR — No effect unless additional +2.50 D spheres are introduced; then stereoacuity improves from 400 sec of arc to 100 sec of arc.*

Improved stereopsis produced by the compensating prisms is a favorable sign (see p. 60).

Parent Consultation

Parents are advised that prognosis for overcoming the strabismus with vision therapy is very good. Prognosis is not at all favorable in regard to eliminating a need for compensatory lenses, but there is no reason to think that contact lenses cannot be used in lieu of spectacles.

A second visit is recommended for additional placement testing.

VISIT 2 (ONE WEEK LATER)

Vectotrainer

(See p. 63.)

Patient reports fusion (a single quoit) when vectograms are positioned to compensate for his esotropia; that is, when they are positioned at 25 PD base out on the instrument scale and he views them without any additional plus lenses before his eyes, or when he views them through additional +2.50 D spheres (OU) and they are positioned on the scale at 10 PD base out. This is an *optimal response.* Patient is uncertain about stereo effect. He thinks he sees some depth but is not sure.

Vergence ranges, measured through additional +2.50 D spheres and compensatory 10 PD base-out lenses: fusion maintained between 0 and 6 PD base out on the instrument scale; beyond those points, fusion breaks down.

Variable-Mirror Stereoscope

(See p. 65.)

Patient reports stereopsis (a single, three-dimensional target) when mirror panels are positioned in accord with his esotropia; that is, when they are positioned at 25 PD base out on the instrument scale and he views them without any additional plus lenses before his eyes, or when he views them through additional +2.50 D. spheres (OU) and they are positioned at 10 PD base out on the scale. This is an *optimal response.*

Vergence ranges, measured through additional +2.50 D spheres and 10 PD compensatory base-out lenses: fusion maintained between 0 and 8 PD base out on the instrument scale.

Anaglyph TV Trainer

(See p. 66.)

Patient reports left eye suppression when he is positioned 6 m from television screen. This response changes to intermittent suppression when compensating 10 PD base-out prism lenses are introduced. This is an *optimal response.*

---

* +2.50 D spheres were used because +3.00 D spheres blurred visual acuity at the 40-cm test distance.

Fusion ranges under these conditions, measured (with a prism bar) as patient wears 10 PD compensatory base-out lenses: binocularity maintained between 0 and 5 PD base out. Tests repeated at 3 m and at 0.5 m. Results much the same as when measured at 6 m.

Prognosis for Remediation Through Vision Therapy

An optimal response was obtained in each of the three tests, Vectotrainer, Variable Mirror-Stereoscope, and Anaglyph TV Trainer (the last at all test distances). In other words, when both of his maculae are stimulated simultaneously by similar stimuli, the patient fuses them and recognizes disparate stimuli within the fused field. Hence, prognosis for vision therapy is very good.

Recommendation

Vision therapy should be successful *if* patient is sufficiently motivated, devotes enough time and effort to the undertaking, and is capable of learning how to alter a habitual visual behavior by exploiting feedback-training principles (see pp. 2–3).

Estimated Time Required

About a year, with most office visits occurring during the first few months of treatment. (Absolute time frames cannot be stated; estimates will be much more accurate once therapy has begun and patient progress can be monitored.)

Patient's Obligations

To devote about 30 to 45 minutes per day at the onset, divided into about three segments.

We stress that treatment will not be a series of muscle exercises; rather, therapy will be designed to teach the patient—or, more accurately, make it possible for him to teach himself—how to obtain and sustain binocular alignment; first by using devices that provide visual feedback signals that he will match up with how it feels when he is using his eyes together in a normal fashion, then by depending upon intrinsic (what-it-feels-like) cues alone.

Patient states that he is very interested. Parents are obviously pleased. We caution them that their child is an adolescent; today's commitment may not be as intense tomorrow. The parents' obligation is to encourage the patient, but not necessarily to coerce him. If his motivation wanes significantly, the treatment will fail. If this does occur, it may be better to delay therapy until he matures a bit. Hence, they have to walk a fine line between wanting him to follow through, recognizing that the final decision is his, and knowing that he is not yet an adult.

Patient is given a new lens prescription—(OU) +5.25 −0.75 cx 180/add +2.50; 5 PD base-out Fresnel prism each eye—and advised to wear them constantly. The laboratory is instructed to position the top of the segs at the lower edge of the patient's pupils.*

No therapy procedures are to be dispensed until after new glasses have been obtained and worn for a while.

---

*See remarks regarding seg placement in case report of patient 4.3. In that situation, the patient was significantly younger and much less self-directed; hence, segs had to be placed very high in the lens. In this case, the patient is more dependable—more likely to follow directions—but more susceptible to being annoyed if segs are too high.

VISIT 3 (ONE MONTH LATER)

Patient has been wearing his new glasses for about two weeks without any apparent difficulty. He is aware of the two powers incorporated into each lens, but it does not bother him at all. He is somewhat annoyed by the Fresnel prisms—"they blur things a little"—but not to a significant degree. Parents report that his eyes appear to be straighter with the new glasses, but they also think his eyes look "worse" (more misaligned) when he takes them off.

Cursory inspection indicates that the segs do, indeed, reduce the deviation and that without them the magnitude of his strabismus is the same as it was before. Parents are informed that what they are observing is caused by the relative effect of the new lenses and that he is no worse. (We should have forewarned the parents of this effect when we dispensed the new lens prescription. This was an oversight of our part.)

On the basis of data derived at the previous visit, patient could start with any one of the three procedures on which he demonstrated binocular potential. We selected procedure 4 (Variable-Mirror Stereoscope) simply because there was one available in the office and the patient seemed to enjoy using it. The procedure was explained and the special-instructions section amended to advise the patient that he was to look at the targets through the segs in his new lenses—at least until he had accomplished substantial improvement in fusional ranges. (We also told him that if he wanted some variation he could attempt to go through the activities again, looking through the distance portion of his lenses. He was cautioned, however, that this would probably be impossible at this beginning stage.)

The next appointment scheduled for two weeks hence.

VISIT 4 (TWO WEEKS LATER)

Patient reports compliance and progress.

Re-administration of placement tests (quoit vectograms, Variable-Mirror Stereoscope, and anaglyph TV Trainer) indicate that his near-point fusional vergence ranges have increased significantly. When measured through the +2.50 D add (OU) and compensating (10 D base-out) Fresnel prisms, he is able to maintain fusion from 10 PD base out to 2 PD base in; however, because he is not yet able to obtain stable fusion without the aid of compensating prisms, he remains in level I of the therapy sequence.

Patient is advised that he has made improvement. He is advised to continue with the same procedure and return in two weeks.

VISIT 5 (TWO WEEKS LATER)

History Update

Patient reports compliance and improvement. He has been able to obtain fusion with the mirrors of the variable-mirror stereoscope set at 6 PD base in on the scale, but only for very brief periods. (This means that at near—with the aid of the additional +2.50 D spheres—he can come within 4 PD of alignment, taking into account the 10 PD base-out Fresnels attached to his present lenses.) He also reports that he thinks he can "fix" his eyes in a way that simulates what he feels with the device, even when he is not using it. This is a major accomplishment.

Re-assessment shows that his vergence ranges within the Variable-Mirror Stereoscope (when measured through his +2.50 D add and the 10 PD base-out Fresnels) now extends from 10 PD base out to 10 PD base in, although he sometimes loses clarity when attempting to meet the demands of the base-in prisms. As such, the patient continues to be placed in level I but is much improved from where he started.

Patient is advised accordingly and questioned about his interest in continuing with same procedure. Patient admits some desire for change. We therefore dispense procedure 16 (red-green stereo trainer). This not only will provide something different but also will enable the patient to continue to develop his newly learned abilities at different fixation distances. We considered reducing the amount of compensating prism in his glasses but decided against it because of the other changes we were making—the shift to a new instrument and the introduction of far-point activities. Too many changes at one time might create some difficulties.

Fusional vergence ranges with stereo trainer measured at the completion of the visit (with prism bar through his compensating prisms):

AT FAR (6 m) 10 PD base out to 4 PD base in
AT NEAR (50 cm) 10 PD base out to 8 PD base in

On the basis of this information, patient is provided with a horizontal prism bar and shown how to position the prisms before his eyes to create the vergence demands that will help him increase fusional ranges and acquire facility. His goal is to be able to perform abrupt fusion jumps from 10 PD base in to 10 PD base out while fixating on a distant target through his present lenses.

Patient advised to return in two weeks.

VISIT 6 (TWO WEEKS LATER)

Patient reports compliance and continued improvement. Through his present lenses, which contain 10 D of compensating base-out prism, he is now able to execute far-point fusional vergence jumps from 10 PD base in to 10 PD base out, and back again, although he has not yet been able to do this with the facility (speed) called for in the printed instructions we gave him. Patient and parents very pleased with his obvious improvement. They believe that his eyes are now straight and inquire about when they can investigate the feasibility of contact lenses. We urge them to allow a bit more time. Contact lenses are, indeed, feasible at this time, but they would necessitate the use of bifocals because of the patient's continued need for prism and additional plus at near. Once explained, this is accepted.

Patient is advised to continue as is, working hard to achieve facility, and, unless something unexpected arises, to return in one month.

VISIT 7 (ONE MONTH LATER)

Patient reports continued compliance and improvement. With the help of the compensating Fresnel prisms, he is now able to execute the 20-PD fusional vergence jumps between 10 PD base in and 10 PD base out within the time constraints called for in his printed instructions. He also reports that he thinks he can keep his eyes straight without the help of the compensating prisms. (He tried the stereo trainer activity with his old glasses, which have no prism, and was able to maintain fusion. He did not persist at this because his parents became anxious about his "doing something wrong.")

Given patient's excellent progress, it is now reasonable to eliminate some of the compensating prism. This is accomplished by removing the 5 PD Fresnel from his left lens and leaving the one on his right lens intact. This has the effect of helping his left eye acuity a trifle, which is to the good inasmuch as that eye is somewhat amblyopic. Patient notices the difference but is not bothered by it.

Patient is advised to continue with same procedure, but to engage in his exercises—to practice fusional vergence jumps with the hand-held prisms—at different distances from the stereo trainer: 6 m, 3 m, 1 m, and so forth. He is also forewarned that because we eliminated 5 D of base-out prism from his lenses the activities will now be somewhat more difficult. He comprehends this. We also reassure him that he is not doing anything harmful when he practices the activities through his old glasses; however, we caution him to limit those experiments to far-point viewing conditions. (Remember, the old glasses have neither compensating prisms nor the extra plus power for near-point conditions.)

Patient asked to return in one month. (Few patients have the self-discipline to maintain a training regimen with such a long time between office visits; however, this patient did, and we took advantage of it.)

VISIT 8 (ONE MONTH LATER)

Patient reports continued improvement. Wearing his glasses, he can execute 22 PD fusional vergence jumps from about 7 PD base in to 15 PD base out and back again with great facility at any distance from the TV Trainer. (Keep in mind that his glasses now provide only 5 PD base-out compensatory prism.) In addition, he is able to maintain fusion through his old glasses (no prism, no extra plus add) from 6 m to about 2 m. When he gets closer than that, fusion breaks down. Hence, the additional plus power for near is still important.

He also tells us that he has been practicing maintaining alignment at other times as well (in the absence of the TV Trainer) and has noted that he is able to detect, in two ways, when his eyes are "working right": (1) He sees double when his eyes are out of alignment—"if he thinks about it." (2) His eyes "feel" different when they are in alignment than when they are not. We attempt to inspire the patient to be more explicit in his descriptions about those "feelings," but he is unable to express them in any concrete way.

Patient is congratulated for his progress and advised to practice his newly learned skills for a while rather than attempt to extend fusional vergence ranges any further at this time. We suggest about 15 to 30 minutes a day with the TV Trainer (both with his new and old glasses) and that he continue to work on gaining fusion without the feedback of the TV Trainer. We also encourage him to think about how he could express more clearly just what he does feel and see when he aligns his eyes and "knows it."

Patient to return in two weeks.

VISIT 9 (TWO WEEKS LATER)

Patient reports increasing self-awareness of his binocular status. He can now maintain alignment whenever and wherever he "thinks about it," and he notes that he can regain fusion almost instantaneously when his strabismus does manifest. (This loss of fusion happens only when he is wearing his old glasses to do some of the activities.) He demonstrates this for us by manifesting his strabismic and aligned postures upon request without much apparent effort. (His normal (i.e., habitual) posture continues to be esotropia when he is not wearing glasses.)

Patient is once again congratulated and advised to continue with the stereo trainer procedure (16), but with stronger prisms. We lend him 5, 10, and 15 D prisms (one each) and show him how to hold them in front of his eyes in combination to practice executing fusional vergence jumps of as great as 25 PD at distance and near—first while wearing his new glasses (the ones with the 5 D base-out Fresnel prism and the extra plus power for near), then with his old ones.

Patient to return in one month.

VISIT 10 (ONE MONTH LATER)

Patient reports continued compliance and improvement. He can execute the fusional vergence jumps we prescribed,although not quite with the desired facility. In addition, he reports that he is now able to maintain fusion with effort using the TV Trainer and his old single-vision, no-prism glasses while standing as close as 2 ft from the stereo trainer.

Our assessment reveals that the patient is able to demonstrate 2 min of arc stereoacuity at far point and 70 sec of arc at near point without the help of compensating prisms. (He did require the extra plus for near to accomplish this.)

We recommend removal of the second Fresnel compensating prism. The patient appears to be able to maintain binocular alignment without this aid under most circumstances and is able to detect a loss of fusion and regain it almost at once when it does occur. In effect, he has just achieved the goals of level I in the constant strabismus therapy sequence. Patient and parents are very pleased.

We also suggest that patient stop daily exercises. He is now at the point where he is practicing binocular alignment just about all the time anyway. There is probably some benefit to be derived from not introducing more prism at this time and from simply giving him time to consolidate his gains.

Patient to return in two weeks.

VISIT 11 (TWO WEEKS LATER)

Patient eager to get back to therapy. He reports no problems. Binocularity is not yet automatic, but it seems to be less of an effort each day.

Our assessment corroborates his observations. He has no need for any compensatory prism. In fact, he is almost able to maintain binocular alignment at near without the aid of the extra plus spheres, although he cannot do this for very long unless he "allows his sight to blur" (i.e., relaxes accommodation).

We recommend that he return to his stereo trainer activities, working mainly at near point, and attempt to perform some of them through the upper portion of his lenses rather than through the segs. In addition, procedure 3-I (eccentric rectangles at near point, no instrument) is explained and dispensed. (We first made sure that he was capable of perceiving physiological diplopia without difficulty.) Patient is instructed to devote about five to ten minutes a day to procedure 3-I, doing it while looking through his segs.

Patient to return in two weeks.

VISIT 12 (TWO WEEKS LATER)

Patient reports that he continues to become more facile at fusional vergence jumps with the stereo trainer at near point. He also states that he has made some progress with procedure 3-I but has not yet accomplished its final goal.

Our assessment confirms his reports. For all practical purposes, patient is no longer a constant strabismic. He has achieved the goals of level III of the constant strabismus therapy sequence (see p. 70) and is now an intermittent (convergence-excess) esotrope; that is, he is almost never strabismic at distance fixation, but he sometimes loses alignment at near, especially when he does not have the support of his segs. As such, patient is now treated according to the guidelines described in chapter 4 and placed on level II of the intermittent-strabismus sequence.

Patient is congratulated and urged to continue the good work. Procedure 3-II is dispensed. Patient is advised to devote less time and effort to the stereo trainer and to work hard on procedures 3-I and 3-II.

Patient to return in two weeks.

VISIT 13 (TWO WEEKS LATER)

Patient reports mastery over procedure 3-I so long as he does the activities through the segs in his glasses. Procedure 3-II is still too demanding, although he finds that he can almost accomplish it when he uses his 5-D prism, base out.

Patient's vergence ranges are starting to approach normal levels. Measured without any compensating prisms they are:

AT FAR From 15 PD base out to 2 PD base in (30 cycles/5 min)

AT NEAR From 16 PD base out to 7 PD base in (45 cycles/5 min)

Patient is advised to continue working on procedures 3-I and 3-II. We also add procedure 3-III to his regimen.

Patient is asked to return in one month.

VISIT 14 (ONE MONTH LATER)

Patient reports mastery over all three parts of procedure 3: he has achieved facility in exercising positive and negative relative convergence using chiastopic and orthopic fusion techniques at distance and near while holding accommodation constant.

Our assessment confirms his report. He is able to achieve the final goal in the intermittent strabismus and vergence facility sequences. For all practical purposes, patient is cured; however, we urge him to practice procedure 3-III for a few minutes each day for the next six months.

Patient is also advised that he has reached the stage where the additional plus power for near (bifocal) may be eliminated. As such, this is a good time to consider replacing his spectacles with contact lenses. In fact, contact lenses are probably preferable at this point in that they will ease the difficulty of the transition from bifocals to single-vision lenses. There are at least three reasons for this: (1) Contact lenses make clear near-point vision possible with less accommodation; (2) contact lenses provide patient with better spatial localization skills because of a more normal image size and larger visual fields; and (3) contact lenses eliminate the induced base-out prismatic effect that strong plus lenses often create.

Patient to return to this office in six months and to phone us before then if problems arise.

VISIT 15 (SEVEN MONTHS LATER)

Patient reports no problems. He has engaged in maintenance activities daily and believes that his eyes are now habitually in alignment. He wants to obtain contact lenses.

Our assessment corroborates his observations (all testing done through distance prescription):

AT FAR	Cover test:	Orthophoria
	Stereoacuity:	1 min of arc
	Vergence facility:	Passes with ease
	Accommodation facility:	Passes with ease
AT NEAR	Cover test:	Orthophoria
	Stereoacuity:	40 sec of arc
	Vergence facility:	Passes with ease
	Accommodation facility:	Passes with ease

(We believe that cover test results—orthophoria—would deteriorate toward esophoria if occlusion was prolonged a few minutes or more. But that is as expected.)

Patient is congratulated for his diligence and success. He is also advised to continue maintenance activities but on a less demanding schedule—about one or two minutes, once or twice per week. (We typically suggest that the patient select times when he is likely to be doing the same thing each week (e.g., getting ready to go to school or church). This should go on for a very long time, thereby assuring the patient that there will be no remissions. (We must acknowledge that this was a remarkable patient; motivated, intelligent, and diligent. We also want to point out that he was at just the right age. Had he been younger, we doubt that he would have been as motivated. We also question whether he would have had the ability to interpret what he was learning from the activities. The point is that it is not always wise to initiate vision therapy with very young patients. As stressed earlier, the activities are not muscle builders; they are lessons that, if effective, teach the patient a new behavior.)

Patient 6.2—Esotropia (Unfavorable Prognosis)

VISIT 1

Patient is a 10-year-old male.

Chief Complaints

He has a long history of right esotropia. Condition initially noted before he was 6 months old. First glasses were prescribed at age 2, used in conjunction with a patch over left eye. Patching discontinued after about six months, at which time patient underwent strabismus surgery. The operation seemed to help, but he still looked a little cross-eyed. The surgeon suggested a second operation when the child was about 5 years old, but because the deviation was not very large, parents rejected the suggestion. Parents are now concerned about "lazy eye"—they recently read an article about amblyopia. They are not very concerned about the child's cosmetic appearance; the untrained observer does not detect the child's strabismus. (Photographs of the child, taken before his strabismus surgery, indicate a significant esotropia, approximately 40 PD.)

Salient Clinical Data

Health status: No evidence of pathology

Visual acuity (unaided): (OD) 20/30; (OS) 20/20

Refractive status: (OU) +0.25 −0.50 cx 90

Binocular status

AT FAR 8 PD constant, comitant, alternating esotropia

AT NEAR 18 PD constant, comitant, alternating esotropia (OS is the preferred eye.)

The above data enable us to determine a preliminary prognosis as follows (see pp. 60–62 and Figure 6.1):

Effect of fixation distance The increase in esotropia occurring when fixation is shifted from distance to near is a *favorable sign.*

Effect of additional +3.00-D spheres (OU) at near Magnitude of deviation does not change noticeably. This is *not* a favorable sign (see p. 66).

Effect of compensating prisms on fusion

AT FAR Patient reports seeing four dots (Worth Dot Test) when tested without glasses and is uncertain about what he sees when compensating prism (20 PD base out) is introduced, thus suggesting ARC; *not* a favorable sign.

AT NEAR Same responses as at far point

Effect of compensating prisms on stereopsis

AT FAR No effect (*not* a favorable sign)

AT NEAR No effect (*not* a favorable sign)

Parent Consultation

Parents are advised that prognosis is not very optimistic, but because we did observe one favorable sign, we recommend a second visit. (Clearly, the apparent ARC response requires that we do keep in check whatever enthusiasm we might feel.) Parents agree to second visit, recognizing that the probability of our recommending vision therapy is slight.

VISIT 2 (ONE WEEK LATER)

Vectotrainer

(See p. 63.)

Patient reports fusion (a single quoit) when vectograms are at the zero position, thus indicating ARC. Testing with this device was stopped.

Variable-Mirror Stereoscope

(See p. 65.)

Patient reports fusion when the mirror panels are at the zero position, again indicating ARC.

Anaglyph TV Trainer

(See p. 66.)

Patient once more demonstrates ARC.

Prognosis for Remediation Through Vision Therapy

Very unfavorable. ARC responses were elicited from all procedures.

Recommendation

Two options were discussed: (1) Referral to an optometrist who specializes in strabismus vision therapy, and (2) reassurance that the child's present visual status is quite stable and that there is no need to be concerned about amblyopia developing beyond its present state. In other words, leave well enough alone.

Parents chose to seek an additional opinion from the specializing optometrist we mentioned to them. That practitioner also dissuaded them from vision therapy. Parents are now satisfied that they have done everything they could, short of another surgical procedure, and have been further assured by us and others that there is no good reason to consider that type of treatment.

Patient 6.3—Accommodative Esotropia (Managed Incorrectly During Early Years)

VISIT 1

Patient is a 7-year-old female who recently obtained glasses from another practitioner.

Chief Complaints

She began almost immediately to manifest exotropia when wearing her glasses. (This was patient's first visit to our office.) History reveals that child had been an esotrope during early childhood, first manifested at about age 18 months. At that time, parent had taken child to the optometrist, who diagnosed accommodative esotropia and strongly recommended glasses for full-time wear. These were obtained and were effective in bringing the eyes into alignment. Parents, however, did not like the way the glasses magnified the child's eyes. After a few months, child was taken to a surgeon who assured the parent that surgery would correct the child's condition. Surgery was performed, and, indeed, child's eyes were straight without glasses. Parents were very pleased.

Upon entering first grade, child started to experience learning problems and ocular discomfort symptoms: headaches, eyestrain, etc. (There had been some hint of this during kindergarten, but not enough to prompt the parents to arrange for an eye examination.) Child was taken for eye examination to a local practitioner, who prescribed (OU) + 7.00 D spheres and explained that lenses were essential. These were obtained and produced exotropia when the child was wearing the glasses. Parents were dismayed and decided to obtain another opinion—hence, the visit to our office.

Salient clinical data

Health status: No evidence of pathology

Visual acuity (without glasses): (OD) 20/70; (OS) 20/70

Visual acuity (with glasses): (OD) 20/30; (OS) 20/30

Refractive status: (OU) + 7.25 D spheres (no significant change from present prescription).

Binocular status

Without prescription

AT FAR 2 PD esophoria

AT NEAR 8 PD esophoria (Patient expressed discomfort at sustaining near fixation.)

With prescription

AT FAR 35 PD constant, comitant left exotropia

AT NEAR 20 PD constant, comitant left exotropia

(Visit took place during late afternoon; mother observed that child's exotropia manifested less consistently during morning hours.)

The above data enable us to determine a preliminary prognosis as follows (see pp. 60–64 and Figure 6.1):

Effect of fixation distance Exotropia (with glasses) decreases significantly when fixation is shifted from distance to near. This is a *favorable sign.*

Effect of additional −3.00 D spheres (OU) at near Deviation reduces to 5-PD intermittent exotropia. This significant reduction in the angle signifies a *favorable sign.*

Effect of compensating prisms on stereopsis

AT FAR Without Rx, patient displays poor stereopsis; targets are too blurred. With Rx, patient reports diplopia.

AT NEAR Same responses as at far; these are *not* favorable signs.

Developmental Status (See chapter 7)

TVAS score = 5 (significantly below expected)
TAAS score = 9 (satisfactory)

The substandard TVAS score did not come as a surprise. Hyperopic children who do not wear compensating lenses during their preschool years often present such a clinical picture.*

Conclusions: This is a unique case but, unfortunately, not as unusual as one would hope. Clearly, the child was an accommodative esotrope who now manifests secondary exotropia when she wears her plus lenses. Yet she has no option but to wear plus lenses if she is to function satisfactorily in school. Hence, the following reasoning process was presented to parent: Child needs plus lenses to see clearly and comfortably; plus lenses cause exotropia, an unacceptable situation; vision therapy could be instituted to help the child acquire the vergence ranges needed to overcome the exotropia, but in our opinion, this is not a sensible undertaking. The task would be much too arduous because of the magnitude of the deviation; the high AC/A ratio; and the child's age, school placement, and significantly delayed visual perceptual skills development.

We therefore suggested a surgical consultation and recommended a pediatric ophthalmologist. We stressed to parent that the surgery would not eliminate the child's hyperopia; she will continue to need lenses. If successful, however, the surgery will allow her to maintain single, simultaneous binocular vision with the lenses in place. This is essential if she is to meet her school requirements. We also advised parent of the child's substandard visual analysis skills but suggested that this concern be put aside until appropriate actions were taken in regard to the strabismus.

Parent not pleased, but accepts recommendation.

VISIT 2 (TWO MONTHS LATER)

History Update

Surgery was conducted about one month ago. Child now wears her glasses; she reports comfortable vision. Mother reports that the youngster's eyes are now straight when glasses are worn, and sometimes crossed when glasses are not worn; however, she now understands the situation and is satisfied that the correct steps have been taken. Mother is interested in obtaining contact lenses as soon as is practical.

Our examinations reveals:

Health status: No evidence of pathology
Visual acuity (without glasses): (OD) 20/70; (OS) 20/70
Visual acuity (with glasses): (OD) 20/30; (OS) 20/30
Refractive status: (OU) +7.25 D spheres
Binocular status

Cover test with Rx

AT FAR Orthophoria
AT NEAR Orthophoria

* For more details and discussion, see J Rosner and J Gruber, Differences in the perceptual skills development of young myopes and hyperopes, *AJOPO* 1985; 62:501–504.

Stereoacuity with Rx

AT FAR 2 min arc

AT NEAR Passes Random-Dot E Stereotest at 1.5 m

Developmental status

TVAS score = 6 (significantly below expected)

TAAS score = 9 (satisfactory)

Conclusions

Child's visual status is now satisfactory. Her hyperopia is appropriately compensated by her glasses and she maintains single, simultaneous binocular vision without effort. (This is not surprising nor is it totally attributable to the second surgical procedure. The child has always had good potential for binocularity. The second surgical procedure made it possible for her to take advantage of that potential.) Her visual analysis skills continue to lag significantly. This should be addressed before the child gets too much further along and further behind in school.

Prescription

Perceptual skills remediation to be administered at home under parent supervision, with her school providing the child with additional structure until her skills have reached the level where such special accommodation is no longer needed.

Parent accepts recommendation; child is now engaged in the remedial program. (See chapter 7 for detailed information about what such a program entails.)

Patient 6.4—Infantile Estropia and Amblyopia

VISIT 1

Patient is a 14-month-old male.

Chief Complaints

Pediatrician and parents have noted strabismus since the child born: "his right eye turned in." Initially they were inclined to wait and see. Now they have become anxious. History revealed a normal pregnancy and delivery (Apgar = 9). There is a familial history of strabismus: two of the child's paternal uncles manifested infantile (congenital) strabismus; neither was treated successfully. At this stage in their lives—even though they are both successful in their respective careers—they and the rest of the family regret that the strabismus was never treated; this because of the cosmetic implications. Neither parent expressed any concern about their child's eyesight. They report that he "likes to look at things" and easily recognizes them from across the room.

Salient Clinical Data

Health status: No evidence of pathology

Visual acuity: We attempted to assess this using a Preferential Looking procedure but were unsuccessful; child's responses were unreliable. We had similar results with the candy-bead procedure. The only useful information obtained was that child was much more resistant to occlusion of his left eye than his right eye. The inference—strongly supported by the apparent unilateral (right) esotropia—is that visual acuity of right eye is significantly worse than visual acuity of left eye.

Refractive status

Dynamic retinoscopy: (OU) +1.50 −0.75 cx 90

Cycloplegic retinoscopy: (OU) +2.00 −0.50 cx 90

Binocular status (Hirschberg test)

40 PD constant, right esotropia; deviation appears to be unaffected by fixation distance. When measured through additional +3.00 D spheres, OU: No change in magnitude of deviation.

Preliminary Prognosis

Not favorable; we did not elicit a single favorable sign. Magnitude of deviation was not affected by fixation distance or by introduction of additional plus spheres. We were unable to assess the effect of compensatory prisms on fusion or stereopsis.

Recommendations

Prognosis for an easy cure is not favorable; however, certain steps should be taken and the situation re-evaluated as the effects of these actions become apparent. Specifically, patching therapy should be instituted at once, using the regimen defined in Table 5.1 (left eye to be patched for three days, then right eye for one day, and so on for the next ten days). (We stress that the patch for this age child must be one that eliminates the possibility of ambient light entering the occluded eye. To accomplish this, we recommend and supply Elastopatch occluders that are applied directly over the child's closed eyelid.) The goal of the recommended treatment is to improve the visual acuity of right eye.

Parents accept treatment recommendations.

VISIT 2 (TEN DAYS LATER)

Parents report that child has gotten used to the patch, although he did "fuss a good bit at first when it was placed over his left eye."

Examination reveals no change in magnitude of deviation; decreased resistance to occlusion of left eye.

Parents are advised that these are favorable indicators, and continuation of patching regimen is recommended.

VISIT 3 (TWO WEEKS LATER)

Parents report no change in child's appearance or attitude toward the patch. (They are disappointed about the former and unemotional about the latter.)

Inspection reveals no change in magnitude of deviation; no significant difference in reaction to occlusion of left eye as compared with right eye.

Cycloplegic refraction is same as on visit 1.

Parents are advised that although there continue to be signs of some improvement in regard to reduction of amblyopia, we see no new favorable signs in respect to the strabismus. We recommend continuation of patching regimen.

VISIT 4 (TWO WEEKS LATER)

Parents report no change.

Inspection reveals no change in magnitude of deviation; deviation unaffected by fixation distance or introduction of additional plus lenses (+3.00 D). Child now manifests an alternating fixation pattern (i.e., he fixates with either eye). There is no change in refractive status measured with cycloplegic. There are no adaptive responses to compensatory prisms, at least in the short-term: 40 PD base out continues to neutralize the strabismus, even after 15 minutes of wear.

We advise parents that patching regimen has worked to the extent that it could. The child no longer appears to be amblyopic. It is now time to discuss next-step options.

1. Put off any further action for a few months. Then re-assess the situation.
2. Prescribe spectacles, not so much to compensate for the moderate refractive error but, rather, as a carrier for prisms that would neutralize the strabismus. The rationale for this is that the use of prisms allows for stimulation of both maculae simultaneously. Thus, if there is any potential for normal binocular function, prisms would be helpful. One potential problem is that the child may adapt to the prisms. This is not a substantial problem, however, in that if it should occur, there would be no long-term effects; it would not make him worse. He would re-adapt to his original state once the prisms were removed. They would simply be a waste.
3. Obtain a surgical opinion.

We reject the first option out of hand. We temper enthusiasm for the second option and suggest strongly that the third option be followed. Parents accept recommendation. We arrange for a consultation with a surgeon who is skillful and patient oriented.

VISIT 5 (THREE WEEKS LATER)

Surgical consultation was obtained about a week ago. We have received report. Parents wish to discuss surgeon's recommendation of strabismus surgery at their convenience within the next month or two.

The surgeon's diagnosis is infantile strabismus: constant, alternating, comitant. No evidence of amblyopia. His prognosis is favorable in respect to cosmesis; guarded in respect to acquisition of central fusion and stereopsis.

We answer parents' questions, explain those aspects of the report that confuse them, and recommend that they follow through with the surgery. In our opinion, given no unfortunate and unforeseen occurrences during surgery, their child's eyes will probably look straight—that is, be within 10 to 15 PD of alignment—and will probably work together satisfactorily albeit not precisely. We also explained the differences between central and peripheral fusion and stereopsis, but we do not think that much of this was understood.

Parents decide to schedule surgery.

VISIT 6 (TWO MONTHS LATER)

Surgery was performed one month ago. Surgeon's report, which was received before this visit, states that treatment was "successful": postoperative state was 10 PD constant, comitant, alternating esotropia. He advised parents to return to us for postoperative care.

Parents appear to be delighted with outcomes from surgery. They perceive their child's eyes to be straight and are anxious only in regard to the long-term prognosis—that is, will the strabismus recur?

Our assessment of the child corroborates what was reported by the surgeon. As such, we advise parents that at this time, there does not appear to be any sign that would indicate that the child is vulnerable to a recurrence of the strabismus. Refraction remains unchanged.

We also advise parents that certain treatment options should now be considered.

1. Child should start to wear glasses that would correct his refractive error and, at the same time, provide sufficient prism to compensate for the residual strabismus. The rationale for this is that the earlier the child begins to experience bifoveal stimulation, the better the chances for ultimate complete rehabilitation.
2. Do nothing now. Re-assess the child's visual status from time to time, and take steps toward further remediation when he is a bit older.

We recommend the first of these. The parents select the second; they do not like the idea of their very young child wearing glasses and, besides, "the operation really worked; his eyes are straight."

VISIT 7 (FIVE MONTHS LATER)

History Update

Parents report no change in child's visual status. His eyes continue to look straight, and he appears to be seeing clearly.

Visual acuity (measured by using a two-item, forced-choice procedure with Allen Picture Card Test): (OD) 20/30−; (OS) 20/30+.

Refraction (measured with cycloplegic): (OD) +2.25 D sphere (20/30); (OS) +2.00 D sphere (20/30+)

Binocular status

Cover test

AT FAR 8 PD esotropia

AT NEAR 12 PD esotropia

Stereopsis (measured without compensating prism, using a modified Frisby stereoacuity test—one that presents only two options, using a forced-choice procedure)*

AT FAR Unreliable responses

AT NEAR 400 sec of arc

* See Gruber and Rosner, Comparison of a modified (two-item) Frisby and RDE stereotests when used with preschool children. AJOPO 1985; 62:349–351.

Prognostic Indications

Effect of additional +3.00 D spheres on magnitude of deviation at near point is negligible.

We inform parents that the options we cited at their last visit are still valid. Their child's eyes are not perfectly straight, even though they certainly look straight. On the other hand, we cannot promise them that lens application and subsequent vision therapy will alter that situation. We also inform them that benign neglect at this time is not very risky; unless something unforeseen occurs, he will never have amblyopia—that is, more than the slight amount he now manifests—nor is it likely that his strabismus will recur.

Parents continue to select the let's-do-nothing-more-at-this-time approach. We accept their decision and advise continued ongoing monitoring. We also tell them that in all likelihood the child will *need* to wear glasses when he begins school, because of his hyperopia and the symptoms it will provoke. In addition, we caution them to provide him with near-point analysis activities to prevent a lag in that aspect of his development.

Child is due to be seen again in this office in about four months. We do not anticipate any major changes in his status and will probably make the same recommendations; however, the final decision regarding this must await that visit.

CHAPTER 7

Perceptual Skills Dysfunction

Perceptual skills dysfunction falls into a category different from the clinical conditions discussed in the five previous chapters. There is no argument about the optometrist's role in the diagnosis and treatment of any of those. There is wide disagreement when it comes to perceptual skills dysfunction, some optometrists contending that it is not within the scope of the profession, others going to the opposite extreme and maintaining that the rubric *perceptual skills* applies to a broad domain of cognitive processes and that the optometrist should occupy a central position in assessment and treatment.

This chapter reflects an in-between perspective based on the propositions that the term *perceptual skills* applies to a very limited and definable set of basic school-learning aptitudes (see glossary, below) and that *all* primary-care optometrists have a fundamental obligation to screen their elementary school–aged patients for perceptual skills dysfunction; explain to the parent, in a nontechnical way, the link between perceptual skills and school performance; report test outcomes, at parental request, to the child's school; and offer appropriate treatment recommendations when a problem is found.

In respect to this last obligation, the suggestions provided in this chapter are guided by the principle that because perceptual skills dysfunction as defined here is primarily an educational problem, the appropriateness of a treatment should be determined on the basis of its likely effect on the child's school performance as well as on his perceptual skills. Improvement of the latter at the expense of the former is often possible but not desirable. The opposite—improvement of the former even to the neglect of the latter—is far more acceptable if, in fact, a choice must be made. (Ideally, of course, there should be no need to neglect one for the sake of the other.) As such, it might be perceived at times that we are arguing against treating perceptual skills dysfunction. That is not the case; rather, we are urging that, if possible, the treatment of perceptual skills dysfunction be coordinated with the other aspects of the child's school program.

GLOSSARY OF TERMS USED IN THIS CHAPTER

This section is included to reduce the confusion that is often created by the lack of a standard vocabulary.

perceptual (analysis) skills* The ability to analyze concrete information in an organized way.

visual perceptual (analysis) skills The ability to analyze spatially organized information in terms of its structural components and to recognize the interrelationships among those components. More specifically, in this context—where achievement in a standard classroom is the main concern—the ability to analyze spatially organized patterns, such as geometric designs, in terms of their concrete (as contrasted with symbolic) features (e.g., the quantity, magnitude, and spatial interrelationships of the separate lines that make up a pattern, rather than the pattern's name or symbolic meaning).

auditory perceptual (analysis) skills The ability to analyze acoustical information in terms of its structural components and to recognize the interrelationships among those components. More specifically, in this context—where achievement in a standard classroom is the main concern—the ability to analyze spoken words in terms of their phonemic (as contrasted with semantic) features (i.e., the separate sounds in a spoken word and the order in which they occur, rather than the word's meaning).

standard classroom A classroom that provides conditions typical of the public schools in the United States; a setting that requires the child to engage in a substantial amount of self-instruction—that is, to learn from cogent examples, application, feedback, self-correction.

A standard classroom consists of (1) an average (by definition) teacher— a person whose knowledge, teaching skills, experience, motivation, energy, and so forth, range from superior to the opposite extreme; (2) a teacher-student ratio of approximately 1:25, thereby requiring group and self-instruction; (3) classes that may or may not be ability grouped (i.e., the class may be homogeneous—made up of children who have been progressing at more or less the same rate; or heterogeneous—comprising a broad range of achievement levels; (4) a finite number of instructional hours per subject per academic year; (5) commercially prepared instructional materials that are designed to be optimally effective with average children; (6) other conditions that limit the amount of individual attention a child can be given.

school achievement The level of school-related skills and knowledge displayed by a child as compared with those displayed by a sample of normal school children of

* The terms *perceptual skills* and *analysis skills* are used here interchangeably. The latter is more accurate, but the former is more popular.

the same grade who were tested in the same way. A separate score is reported for each school subject (reading, arithmetic, spelling, etc.); often, these are broken down into subskills (reading comprehension, word analysis skills, etc.).

Scores are usually reported in terms of grade equivalent (GE), with the numeral to the left of the decimal point representing the grade, that is, year, and those to the right, the month within grade. Thus, GE = 3.2 means that the child performed at a level characteristic of a normal child in the second month of the third grade. Scores may also be reported in percentiles and stanines, but never to the exclusion of the grade equivalent.

intelligence quotient (IQ) An index that purports to predict how well a child will learn in a standard classroom. Most IQ tests are made up of a number of different tasks, each intended to sample from some aspect of cognitive ability. Some items are designed to assess the child's general knowledge level, factual information he has acquired since birth (e.g., vocabulary, number facts, and familiarity with the things—animals, objects, etc.—that exist in the world). Hence, performance in these tends to reflect the child's life experiences to date; they are culture related. Other items are less dependent upon specific knowledge and past experiences; they probe the child's general ability to solve problems, which, to a great extent, depends upon spatial reasoning rather than acquired knowledge—for example, assembling jigsaw puzzles, reproducing block designs, and copying geometric designs.

To arrive at an IQ, the child's responses to these different activities are summed, then compared with what other children of the same age have been able to do with those same tasks. This yields a mental age that is then juxtaposed to the child's chronological age and converted to a standard score—an IQ—wherein 100 represents the average, and the so-called normal range extends from about 90, at the low end, to 110.

In application, the child whose IQ is 100 is expected to learn at an average rate in a standard classroom. The child whose IQ is above 100 is expected to make better-than-average progress; the child with an IQ below 100, the opposite.

underachiever A child whose school achievement does not meet the predictions of his IQ; considering his potential, he is not progressing at the rate one would expect.

overachiever A child whose school achievement exceeds the predictions of his IQ; considering his potential, he is progressing better than one would expect.

academic potential A misconception that has become so well established that it is rarely questioned. Literally, the word *potential* means "something that can develop or become actual."* It implies a limit. In fact, however, the IQ test does not measure potential. As described above, it compares a child with normal children of the same age in two areas that strongly influence school achievement in a standard classroom: how much factual information about the world he has acquired since birth, and how good he is at solving problems that do not depend so much on acquired knowledge as on the general ability to employ spatial reasoning processes. As such, the IQ test does a fair job of predicting how well a child will

* *Webster's New Collegiate Dictionary*, s.v. "potential."

progress in a standard instructional setting, but it hardly approximates an assessment of a child's potential to learn. Presumably, each of us has a finite potential for learning, but the instrument for measuring it has yet to be produced.

SPECIFIC RELATIONSHIPS BETWEEN PERCEPTUAL SKILLS AND SCHOOL PERFORMANCE

Visual and auditory analysis skills are developed, and their rates of development are reasonably predictable. They are the product of normal maturation and early experiences; special lessons are not required. Some children, however, do not develop these skills on schedule, yet they enter first grade in the September following their sixth birthday, ready or not. The outcome is that they are introduced to reading, spelling, writing, and arithmetic—the communication systems of the classroom—before they have acquired the ability to recognize that the information they look at and listen to not only has meaning but also consists of graphic and acoustical (concrete) sensations that, themselves, have very specific characteristics.

Thus exists the connection between perceptual skills and school achievement. Perceptual skills enable the child to identify the concrete, or sensory, features in visual and oral information that the classroom coding symbols code—letters symbolizing the phonemic features (sounds) of spoken language, numerals symbolizing the organizational features (quantity, magnitude, and relationships) of spatial data.

If a child's perceptual skills are deficient, the coding systems he is expected to learn will not make sense. He will not be able to comprehend and employ the association strategies that facilitate learning; he will not recognize how what he already knows can help him remember new, related information. His only alternative in these circumstances is rote memorization of what appears to him to be separate, unrelated facts, an approach that cannot succeed over the long term. The burden is too great; there is too much to learn and remember. School failure is virtually guaranteed.

Visual Perceptual Skills and School Learning

The child with substandard visual analysis skills tends to deal with information, be it written or spoken, in a disorganized way. In general terms, this is most apparent in how he follows directions and completes paper-and-pencil tasks and, more specifically, in the difficulties he encounters in primary-grade arithmetic and reading comprehension.

Arithmetic. Satisfactory progress in arithmetic depends upon the child's capacity to (1) understand and apply the basic algorithms of addition, subtraction, multiplication, and division in the solution of calculation problems; (2) remember a basic set of number facts, thus bypassing the need to recalculate them each time; and (3) apply these remembered number facts in the solution of more complex calculations, thereby reducing the number of steps required to arrive at an answer. The child with visual analysis skills dysfunction, by definition, is not as adept as he should be in identifying the spatial features of quantity, magnitude, and interrelationships—the features that numerals code. As such, the child will not apply the number facts he already knows to the acquisition of additional number facts. Knowing that 2 + 2 = 4 will not facilitate his remembering that 2 + 3 = 5. Rather than recognizing the latter as being a closely associated fact—just one more—he will view it as something completely separate, something to be remembered on its own, as though it were yet another word in a foreign language he is trying to learn. This is hardly an efficient way to learn all the basic number facts that are needed to acquire fluency in arithmetic calculations. True, one unique feature of arithmetic is that one can always figure out the answer to a problem; nothing need be memorized. But practically speaking, figuring it out only works in the primary grades. From about the third grade on, the child has to be able to apply number facts as he does calculations if he is to meet the time requirements of the classroom.

Reading Comprehension. Reading comprehension depends upon two fundamental abilities: one, the ability to convert the printed word to its oral form; the second, the ability to remember the information contained within those words. The first of these—often referred to as word recognition skills—is not closely related to visual analysis skills, but the second is. The child who shows a deficit in the ability to analyze concrete information in an organized way (as demonstrated in his responses to visual perceptual skills tests) usually has similar difficulty analyzing and organizing abstract information such as is contained in printed matter. This, in turn, hampers his ability to retain the information, which then inevitably leads to substandard reading comprehension. This same problem also affects a child's ability to remember spoken information. It is not the sensory modality that counts; it is the general inability to organize information for retention (see additional mention of this in the questions and answers on p. 107).

Auditory Perceptual Skills and School Learning

Auditory perceptual skills have been shown to be closely related to the aforementioned word recognition skills. The 6-year-old with inadequate auditory analysis skills is, by definition, inept at isolating single sounds within the context of spoken words. As such, the system that underlies reading and, to some extent, spelling will be obscure to him. Indeed, if his visual analysis skills are adequate, he will learn to identify the different letters; he will even learn to recognize a short list of words on sight. But he will encounter reading problems fairly early in the primary grades because of his inability to use what he already knows to extend his list of sight words. That he has learned to recognize the word *cat* on sight will not make it easier for him to remember *fat* or *hat*. They will be unrelated, independent facts. The associations between *cat*, *fat*, and *hat* will not be apparent because, although the cogent similarities and differences in their spelling may be noticed, the related similarities and differences in their spoken sounds will not. The child will have to resort to rote memorization, a very unsatisfactory method for learning to read.

IDENTIFICATION

Signs and Symptoms

Not all of the following are displayed or experienced by all patients.

1. Unsatisfactory achievement in the fundamental school subjects—reading, spelling, arithmetic, and writing—that cannot be explained on the basis of the child's physical or emotional states or his IQ. Some children have difficulty in one subject only; some in more than one.
2. Hyperactivity and distractibility, especially when the child is in a standard classroom setting.
3. Inadequate ability to recall (spoken or written) instructions.
4. Reversal errors while reading or printing.
5. Poor spelling skills.
6. Loses place often when copying from chalkboard or book.
7. Sloppy penmanship and paperwork.
8. Difficulty completing written assignments within reasonable time limits.
9. Generally disorganized in work habits, appearance, actions, and the like.
10. A history of premature or other abnormal birth circumstances.
11. A history of delay in one or more aspects of development.

Prevalence

Manifests in approximately 10 to 25 percent of elementary school–aged children, with the variance reflecting how the condition was defined and identified.

Screening Tests

Two types of screening tests are described below; one to detect visual perceptual skills dysfunction, the other, auditory perceptual skills dysfunction.

To Detect Visual Perceptual Skills Dysfunction

The test described below is but one of many that can be used for assessing a child's visual perceptual skills. Also useful are the Rutgers Drawing Test; the Developmental Test of Visual-Motor Integration; the Slosson Drawing Coordination Test; and the Bender Visual-Motor Gestalt Test for Children (all are cited in the bibliography). They all involve copying geometric designs. Each test has its unique characteristics, but in general, the child who performs satisfactorily or unsatisfactorily for his age on any one will do similarly on all the others. Each has been designed and standardized on the strength of the well-documented observation that as children grow and develop they can be expected to become better at performing various tasks that require the analysis of spatially organized patterns, including the copying of geometric designs of increasing complexity. (There also are tests that require behaviors other than the copying of geometric designs, but there is no practical reason to cite them here.)

The Test of Visual Analysis Skills (*TVAS*). The 18 items of this copying test are shown in Figure 7.1 in reduced form.* It can be administered by an office assistant in about five to ten minutes.

1. With children in first grade and below, use response form A (Figure 7.2). This 8½ × 11-in sheet of paper contains spaces for the first 12 items of the test. Typically, children of that age or grade will not proceed beyond item 12.

With children in second grade and beyond, use response form B (Figure 7.3). It contains spaces for the last 12 items of the test (items 7–18), this on the assumption that children beyond first grade rarely have difficulty with the first 6 items.

If these expectations are not upheld in a given instance, simply alter the guideline. In other words, if a first-grade child successfully copies the first 12 items of the TVAS, and if testing is to continue (not essential if the test is being used only for screening purposes), give him form B, locate the response space for item 13 (halfway down the page), and administer the subsequent items. Similarly, if a second-grade child cannot accurately copy item 7, remove form B (without overt or implied criticism), give him form A, and recommence testing with item 1.

2. Seat the child at an appropriately sized table, give him a pencil with an eraser, present the first item he is to copy (item 1 if form A is used, 7 for form B), and say, "*Copy this, here.*" (Point first to model, then to proper space on response form.) "*Make yours look like mine.*" (There are no restrictions on how the directions are stated, so long as the examiner does not show the child how to accomplish the task—for example, where to start, what to do next. Also, there are no restrictions on erasures or on time. If, however, the child is inclined to rush through the activity, thereby performing inadequately, ask him to slow down; conversely, if the child spends an inordinate amount of time on each item in an attempt to be precise, reassure him that it need not be perfect and urge him to move along a little faster.)

3. Continue in this manner until the child has either failed two items in succession or successfully completed item 9. (An item is "passed" if the child draws the correct number of lines and locates them, with reasonable accuracy, on the correct dots. An incorrect number of lines or an incorrect placement on the map—that is, on the wrong dots—constitutes an error, a "failed" item. Neatness is *not* a factor as long as the child shows the abilities just described.)

4. If the child gets to item 10, change the instructions to, "*Now some of the dots are missing from your map; don't draw in the dots; pretend they are there and draw the lines as though the dots were there.*"

* Full-sized versions of these are included in the Procedures manual.

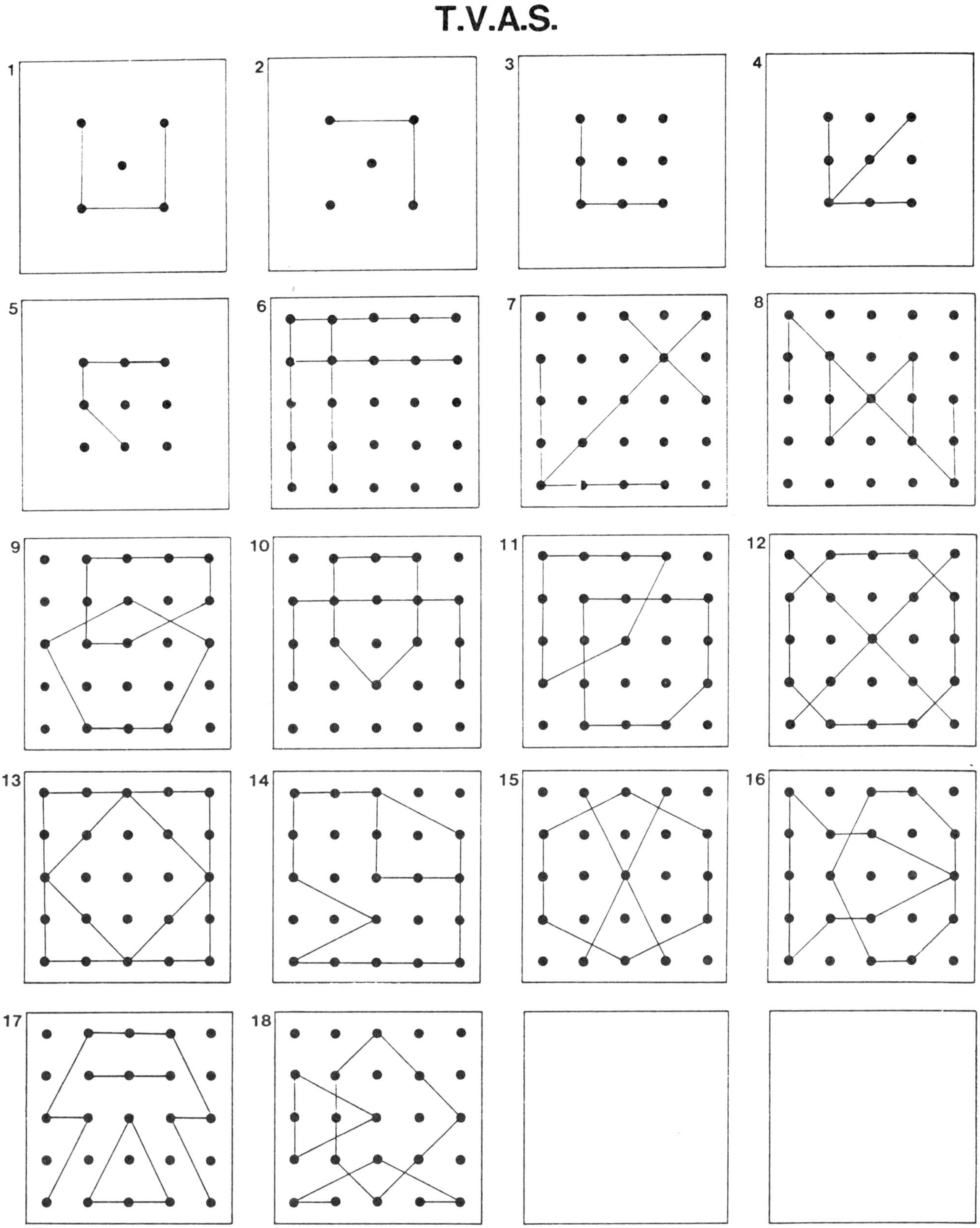

FIGURE 7.1 Test of Visual Analysis Skills (TVAS)

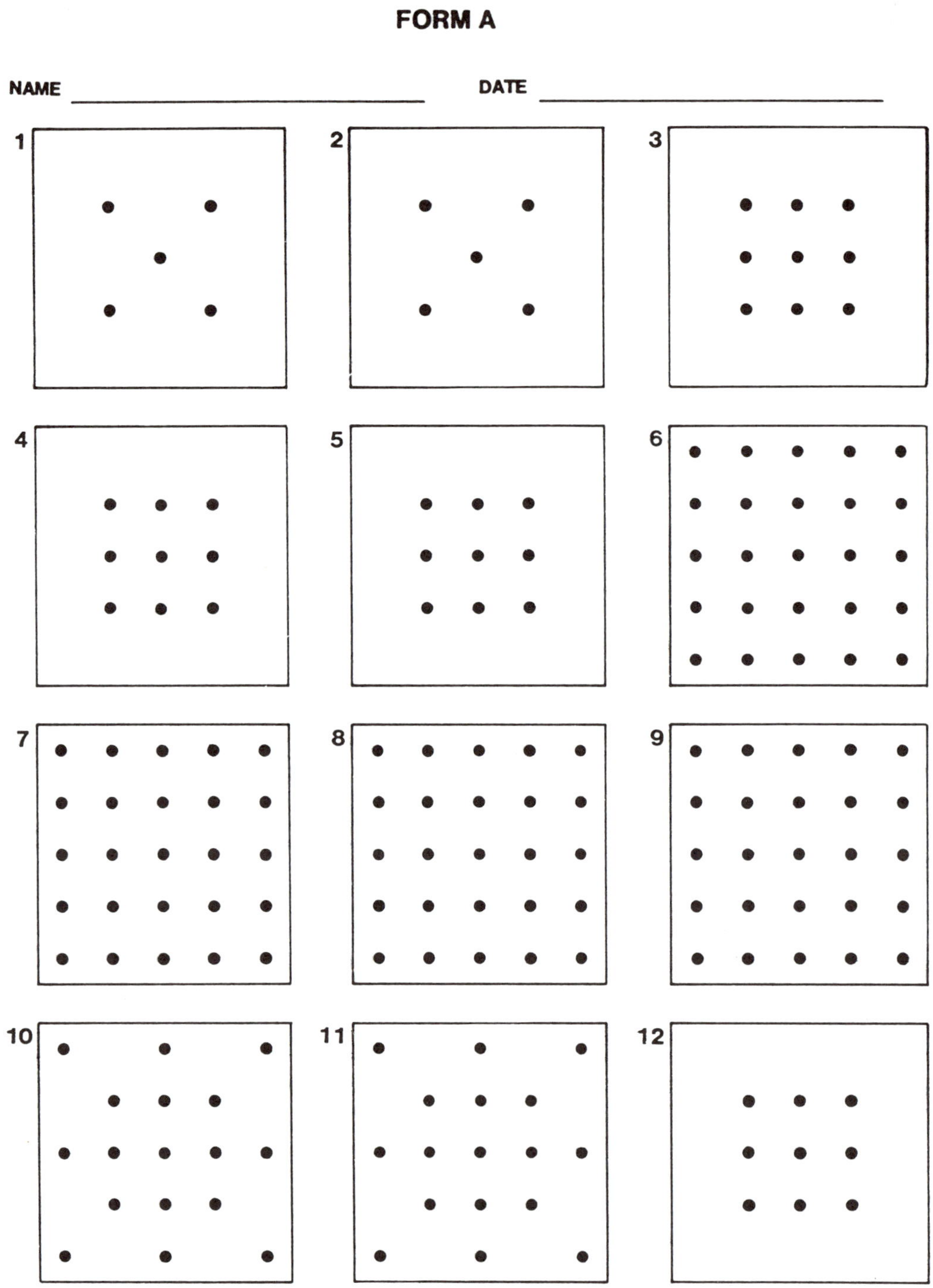

FIGURE 7.2 TVAS Response Form A

FORM B

NAME ______________________ DATE ______________________

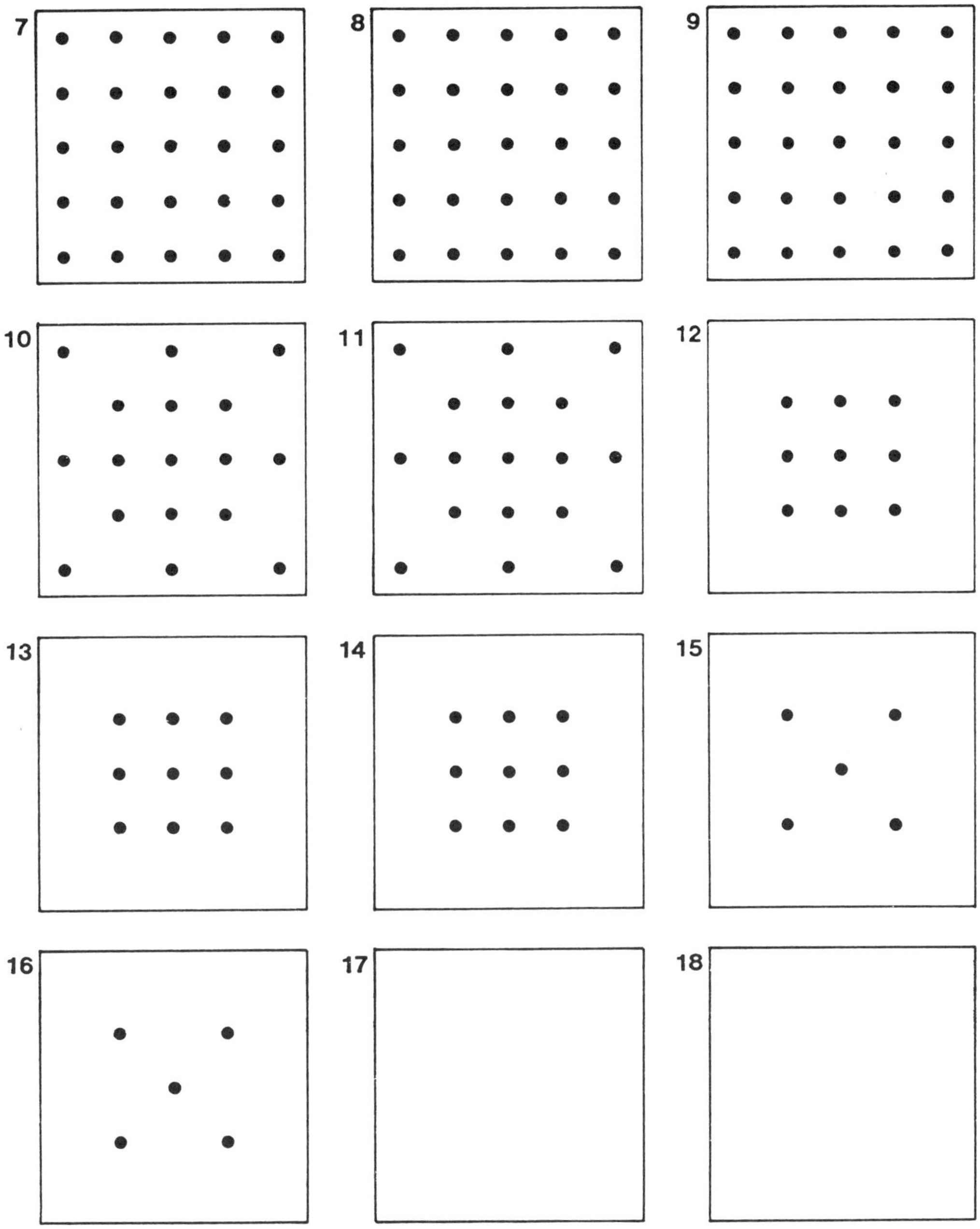

FIGURE 7.3 TVAS Response Form B

5. Continue in this manner until (a) the child goes beyond the level expected for his age, or (b) all 18 items have been completed, or (c) 2 successive items are failed—whichever occurs first.

To score: The TVAS score is the number of the last successfully completed item. Say, for example, that the child passes items 1 through 8, fails item 9, passes item 10, then fails items 11 and 12. The test terminates there (two successive "fails"); his score is 10, the number of the last item passed.

Performance criteria: To determine whether the child's performance is appropriate for his grade placement, consult Table 7.1 where grade level expectations are shown.

QUESTIONS AND ANSWERS ABOUT VISUAL PERCEPTUAL SKILLS

Certain questions often arise at this point in an evaluation.

Q. Does this one test (TVAS) provide enough information to make a valid judgment of the child's visual perceptual skills?

A. Yes. The TVAS provides the information needed to answer the question, Does the child manifest perceptual skills dysfunction? True, a different test might yield somewhat different results, but, except for preschoolers, not different enough to justify their use.

Q. Are printing and reading reversals caused by visual perceptual skills dysfunction?

A. Yes, in many cases; however, this does not mean that the child with persistent reversal tendencies will also demonstrate deficient visual analysis skills when tested with the TVAS. It is altogether possible that the reversal tendencies stem from having been taught the letters at an earlier time, when his visual analysis skills were not yet sufficiently developed to enable him to learn them securely. Often in those instances, the child develops an inefficient strategy for remembering, for instance, the *b* or the *d*, which he then continues to use. It is very possible that since then his visual analysis skills have emerged—he grew out of the problem—but the reversal tendencies remain, an undesirable behavior that has been practiced so long that it becomes established as a bad habit and will remain a habit until someone teaches the child a different (and a better) one.

Q. Do children with visual perceptual skills dysfunction usually grow out of their problem?

A. Yes, most do. But as noted above, that does not mean that they also grow out of the academic problems that were produced because of the poor visual analysis skills. These are likely to remain unless something is done about them.

Q. Does poor performance on the TVAS indicate distorted vision?

A. No. An inadequate response to the TVAS, or any other copying test, does not indicate that the child literally perceives the stimulus in some distorted way.

TABLE 7.1 TVAS Score Expectations

TVAS Score	Expected for children in
1	Preschool
2	Preschool
3	Kindergarten
4	Kindergarten
5	Kindergarten
6	Kindergarten
7	Kindergarten
8	Grade 1
9	Grade 1
10	Grade 1
11	Grade 2
12	Grade 2
13	Grade 2
14	Grade 2
15	Grade 2
16	Grade 2
17	Grade 3
18	Grade 3

This can be easily demonstrated. Show the child two copies of the same pattern—the one he drew that was incorrect and a correct one—and have him identify (point to) the correct one. The majority of the children will match the pattern correctly, evidence that they perceive it correctly. Their problem arises when they are required to duplicate patterns, an activity that involves much more detailed, precise analysis. We all have had analogous experiences. Each of us, at one time or another, has attempted to draw a scene, a person, or an object and has not succeeded very well. This hardly indicates that we could not perceive it accurately.

Q. Does poor performance on the TVAS indicate a fine-motor-skills deficit?

A. No. It is true that teachers often refer children to the optometrist on suspicion of visual perceptual skills dysfunction and send along observations about the child's inept fine motor skills. This probably stems from the false notion that perceptual skills are derived from the child's fine motor skills, which, in turn, emerge from the child's gross-motor-skills development. Hence, the incorrect reasoning is that the child's basic problem lies with his motor skills. In fact, this is very rarely the case.

Q. How then does one differentiate between inept fine motor skills and inadequate visual analysis skills as factors that affect a child's performance on the TVAS or on any other copying test?

A. The simplest method is to reduce the copying test to a fine-motor-skills activity by relieving the child of the responsibility for analyzing the design in terms of its separate components and mapping out their interrelationships. To do this, have the child repeat the first item he failed in the TVAS, but this time, you select a single line in the model and ask the child to *"draw this line from here to here."* (Point in sequence to the two dots that are to be connected by the line.) Then identify a second line and show him where on his map to draw it, and so forth. In other words, you take on the task of singling out each line, one at a time, and locating it on the map of dots. The child's only requirement is to draw the lines, to execute the fine motor actions. Very few children have trouble with this, even though they could not copy the same design under standard TVAS conditions. Those few who do have trouble are the ones whose inadequate performance on the TVAS may be due to poor fine motor skills. The others are more accurately described as lacking in visual analysis skills.

Q. Preschool teachers are becoming increasingly sensitive to perceptual skills dysfunction among three- and four-year-olds. Will the TVAS identify them?

A. It may. The TVAS frequently falls short with children younger than 5. In fact, there are very few performance tests that do consistently work well with that age group. First of all, preschool children are notoriously unreliable test takers. Hence, substandard performance may not be indicative of a problem; it may merely be evidence of the child's capricious attitude about tests. Second, preschool children have very limited capacity to analyze spatially organized patterns and an equally limited repertoire of response abilities. This markedly restricts the number of ways in which they can be tested. There are, however, two easily administered tests that are appropriate for this age group: one is the Gesell Copy Form Test;* the other, the fine motor–adaptive section of the Denver Developmental Screening Test (DDST).† Both investigate the child's ability to copy simple geometric designs, for example, circle, square, plus sign. The Gesell test was designed for children through age 7; the DDST, for children between birth and 6 years. The former has more designs than the DDST, but it does not provide as good a scoring system. All else being equal, the DDST is probably a better test for preschoolers.

Q. Should the child's ability to discriminate figure from ground be tested? Does not this ability influence performance on the TVAS?

A. The answer to both questions is no. Good visual analysis skills are fundamental to the acquisition of good figure-ground discrimination skills, not the reverse. Good figure-ground discrimination skills depend upon one's ability to seek out salient features that are embedded in a distracting background. The capacity to seek out salient features is simply another way of defining perceptual skills.

Q. How is visual memory related to visual perceptual skills?

A. Like figure-ground discrimination, good visual memory depends upon competent visual analysis skills and the ability to generate effective mnemonic strategies. The latter, to a great extent, depends upon being able to identify and label salient features in a way that is memorable. Clearly, then, visual memory is derived from visual perceptual skills in combination with factual knowledge that the child has acquired from previous experiences.

* This test is described in FL Ilg and LB Ames, *School readiness* (New York: Harper & Row, 1965).

† Available from DDM, P.O. Box 20037, Denver, CO 80220.

To Detect Auditory Perceptual Skills Dysfunction

Screening for auditory analysis skills dysfunction parallels what has already been said about visual analysis skills. Developmental studies have shown that as a child matures he becomes more aware of the different sounds in his world—what is most relevant in a discussion of school-related performance is that he becomes aware of the separate sounds in spoken words, recognizing that spoken words are made up of sounds that occur in a specific temporal sequence. Just as with visual analysis skills, this awareness develops on a predictable schedule. At about age 4, the average child shows an awareness of the separate syllables in spoken, two-syllable compound words; then, at age 5, nonmeaningful syllables in polysyllabic words; then, a year or so later, the beginning (single) sound of a spoken word, then the final sound, and so on.

There are not many tests for screening auditory analysis skills, and some of these are less useful than others. Representative of the former are tests that examine the child's ability to discriminate nonverbal sounds (taps, musical sounds, etc.). Somewhat better are tests that assess the child's ability to differentiate between pairs of spoken words that may or may not be the same (e.g., *pen/pin, man/man, boy/toy*). Such tests focus on an important skill, but they do not go far enough, considering the reason for administering a screening test. (Recall the illustration used to explain why copying geometric designs is much more demanding than discriminating similarities and differences. See p. 102. The same is true of auditory processes.)

The test described below requires that the child delete a specified sound from a spoken word. It gets closer than discrimination tests in assessing an aptitude that is fundamental to learning to read. It can be administered by an office assistant in about one or two minutes, and like the TVAS described above, it allows for a comparison of the child's performance with what is typically expected from children of his grade level.

The Test of Auditory Analysis Skills (*TAAS*). This 13-item test is shown in Figure 7.4. No other materials are needed.

1. Figure 7.4 shows items 1 through 13 preceded by two demonstrator items designated *A* and *B*.
2. Present the demonstrator items first. Say to the child, *"Say cowboy; now say it again, but don't say* [*leave off*] boy." Because items A and B are demonstrators, they may be explained to the child if he is confused by the task. However, if a brief explanation does not clear up the confusion, then it is best to stop the test and record a score of zero. The majority of kindergarten children will not be confused by the demonstrator items.
3. If the child shows an understanding of the task (with items A and B), go on to item 1. Here, the syllable is the unit of analysis, as is the case with the next two items as well.
4. If item 4 is reached, a change takes place. At this point, the child is required to delete a single sound. When administering these items, the examiner should state the letter sound, not the letter name. For example, in item 4, after the child has repeated the word *coat*, he is asked to *"Say it again, but don't say*

FIGURE 7.4 Test of Auditory Analysis Skills (TAAS)

A. Say cowboy	Now say it again, but don't say boy	cow
B. Say steamboat	Now say it again, but don't say steam	boat
1. Say sunshine	Now say it again, but don't say shine	sun
2. Say picnic	Now say it again, but don't say pic	nic
3. Say cucumber	Now say it again, but don't say cu(q)	cumber
4. Say coat	Now say it again, but don't say /k/[1]	oat
5. Say meat	Now say it again, but don't say /m/[2]	eat
6. Say take	Now say it again, but don't say /t/[3]	ache
7. Say game	Now say it again, but don't say /m/	gay
8. Say wrote	Now say it again, but don't say /t/	row
9. Say please	Now say it again, but don't say /z/	plea
10. Say clap	Now say it again, but don't say /k/	lap
11. Say play	Now say it again, but don't say /p/	lay
12. Say stale	Now say it again, but don't say /t/	sale
13. Say smack	Now say it again, but don't say /m/	sack

[1] The k sound
[2] The m sound
[3] The t sound

/k/." The parallel slashes (*//*) indicate that the letter sound is to be stated, not the letter name.

5. Stop testing when the child completes the test or fails two successive items, whichever comes first.

To score: The TAAS score is the number of the last item passed. For example, say the child passes items 1, 2, and 3, fails item 4, passes 5 and 6, then fails both 7 and 8. His score is 6.

Performance criteria: To scale a TAAS score, consult Table 7.2, where TAAS grade level expectations are shown.

QUESTIONS AND ANSWERS ABOUT AUDITORY PERCEPTUAL SKILLS

Certain questions are often asked at this point in an evaluation.

Q. Does inadequate performance on the TAAS indicate impaired hearing?

A. Not necessarily, but it might. It is always worthwhile to have the child's hearing tested, just as it is important to have the child undergo a thorough vision evaluation.

Q. Is there any connection between inept auditory analysis skills and a history of frequent ear infections during the preschool years? If there is such a connection, what are the treatment implications?

A. In answer to the first question, yes, many children with auditory analysis skills dysfunction have a history of sporadic ear infections during their early years,

TABLE 7.2 TAAS Score Expectations

TAAS Score	Expected for children in
1	Kindergarten
2	Kindergarten
3	Kindergarten
4	Grade 1
5	Grade 1
6	Grade 1
7	Grade 1
8	Grade 1
9	Grade 1
10	Grade 2
11	Grade 2
12	Grade 3
13	Grade 3

accompanied by episodes of impaired hearing. The treatment implications, however, are the same for them as for other children.

Q. The child has trouble remembering spoken instructions that extend beyond a single, short phrase. Does that indicate substandard auditory analysis skills?

A. No. The child's memory difficulties should not be attributed to inadequate auditory analysis skills. Rather, it is probably because (1) he is not paying attention to the speaker, (2) he is unfamiliar with the words or the topic they pertain to, or (3) the information being expressed is too extensive for him to organize efficiently for storage in short-term memory. If it is the last, suspect visual analysis skills dysfunction, not auditory, even though the information is spoken and heard.

Q. Do children with auditory perceptual skills dysfunction grow out of their problem in time?

A. Yes. But, as with visual analysis skills, that does not mean that they also grow out of the academic problem that was produced because of the poor auditory analysis skills. Unless the academic problem is dealt with successfully, it is likely to persist.

TREATMENT

Factors the Optometrist Should Consider

Prognosis for Remediation Through Vision Therapy.
Generally speaking, prognosis is very favorable, so long as the condition does not stem from organic factors (e.g., CNS involvement). Remedial treatment is far less effective in those cases.

Unfortunately, however, a prognosis is not always that clear-cut; it is not simply a case of whether the perceptual skills dysfunction can be remediated. One must also take into account the effect of the treatment on the problem that is of primary concern to parent and school—the child's unsatisfactory classroom performance, something that the optometrist does not diagnose and treat. This complicates matters.

Three basic facts should be kept in mind when determining prognosis.

Perceptual skills are not the equivalent of acquired knowledge. Rather, they are developed aptitudes that influence how easily a child acquires knowledge (learns) in a standard classroom. They have much less impact in other, out-of-school environments, so long as learning or knowing how to read, write, spell, and calculate is not required.

School achievement is influenced by many factors in addition to perceptual skills. Foremost among these is the child's knowledge state, the extent to which he has or has not learned what his current school lessons presume he knows. Hence, a poor start in the early grades will have compounding detrimental effects on subsequent school achievement, regardless of the original cause.

Therefore, although substandard perceptual skills can often be improved through appropriate treatment, this does not guarantee improved school performance. The child's knowledge deficit—the information he should have but did not learn in earlier grades—will remain until it, too, is eliminated through teaching or self-instruction. If that knowledge deficit is significant, its effect on subsequent school achievement will also be significant, regardless of how improved the perceptual skills. As such, improving the perceptual skills of a fourth- or fifth-grade child who is performing at the second- or third-grade level, and doing nothing else for him, is analogous to hoping—unjustifiably— for a spontaneous improvement in the school performance of a child who, because of illness, did not begin to attend classes regularly until he was 10 years old, at which time he was enrolled in the fifth grade. His health and school attendance record may now be excellent, but if he never learned the basic skills and knowledge of the earlier grades, he will still have to do so.

For these reasons, when formulating a prognosis in respect to the probable outcomes of perceptual skills therapy, the optometrist should take the child's present age and school achievement level into account. He or she must recognize that the child who is already well along and well behind in school will need more than improved perceptual skills in order to satisfy school achievement requirements. He will also need special, nonstandard, appropriately designed, compensatory classroom conditions that make it possible for him to learn despite his current status—a better-than-average teacher who has acquired skills beyond what standard teacher preparation provides, a classroom with fewer children, more precisely defined instructional methods and materials, help and time in organizing his work, and so on. On the other hand, remediating the perceptual skills deficits of a first- or second-grade child who is not yet very far behind in classroom work is very likely to have strong positive effects on school performance.

Alternative Treatment Options

Reassurance This treatment is appropriate only when the patient's perceptual skills are found to be adequate for his age and grade. In such cases, if unsatisfactory school performance is a chief concern, the optometrist's responsibilities are fulfilled when he or she informs the parents of the examination outcomes and urges them to devote their resources to investigating other possibilities, for example, the child's physical status, his emotional state, or—probably most important—his lack of school knowledge, the result of substandard instruction or learning in the lower grades. This latter circumstance is not uncommon and can occur from a variety of causes: poor teaching, for example, or frequent changes of residence that required the child also to change schools while in the primary grades. Schools often differ in when and how certain things are taught, even though, eventually, they all reach the same major instructional goals. The child who is moved from one school to another during those early years runs the risk of missing certain important instructional experiences because of timing mismatches.

It is, of course, also possible that the child did manifest a perceptual skills deficit at one time, and in fact, this may have generated his original learning problems. But speculating about what once may have existed is nonproductive at this point. The practical matter of fact is that he does have a learning problem and does not have a perceptual skills deficit at the present time.

It is also conceivable that one would want to consider reassurance for the child whose perceptual skills disorder is but one small problem among many—for instance, the child who has multiple handicaps, mental retardation, CNS involvement. But, in fact, compensatory treatment is far more appropriate for them than is reassurance.

Referral This option is one that should be exercised regularly by those optometrists who screen for perceptual skills dysfunction but, having identified it, then shy away from offering treatment suggestions.

The best referral for this child depends upon what resources are available in the community. It could be to an optometric colleague who offers such services, to a speech and language specialist, a special education teacher, a psychologist, a child development specialist, or anyone else who knows how to foster the improvement of lagging perceptual skills and is willing to offer his or her services at reasonable cost. When there is uncertainty about the relative quality of available community resources, the parent should be advised to contact the nearest chapter of the Association for Children with Learning Disabilities (ACLD). It is an international organization made up of interested parents and professionals. There are chapters listed in the telephone book all over the United States, and in general, the members are well aware of the resources in their communities. They have learned the hard way, and they are always willing to share what they know.*

* Recently, some school systems have begun to assume responsibility for administering perceptual skills therapy programs, often in collaboration with the optometrist who initially diagnosed the problem. This can be an optimal situation and should be encouraged.

Compensation Compensatory treatment for children with perceptual skills dysfunction means providing the child with instructional conditions that accommodate his existing deficits while, at the same time and as time and energy allow, attempting to remediate the dysfunction.

As explained above, compensatory treatment is probably the best choice for the patient who is beyond third grade and significantly behind in classroom achievement—not because remedial treatment would fail but, rather, because in those situations, remediating perceptual skills dysfunction and doing nothing else will not improve the child's school performance very much. And it is school performance that should be given primary attention, keeping in mind that each day the child slips further behind in what he should know and becomes harder to teach in a standard classroom.

It is not the optometrist's responsibility to define the compensatory instructional conditions; that prerogative belongs to the educator. Certain general guidelines do apply, however, and it behooves the optometrist to be familiar with them so that he or she will be able to offer helpful suggestions to parent and school. On the whole, schools will be responsive if for no other reason than that a federal law (PL 94–142) mandates it.

Unfortunately, some school systems deny any responsibility for providing special help to such children. This is a diminishing problem, but it does exist in certain regions. In those instances, the parent has three options, none of which is very good: (1) Accept the situation, much to the child's detriment; (2) retain a lawyer who will remind the school of its responsibilities, as mandated by federal law; or (3) seek out a private agency (tutor, school, etc.) to provide to the child what he requires for a fee. The first of these is completely unacceptable; the second, expensive in both money and, worse yet, time; the third, expensive—if even available. Here, again, the parent may obtain useful assistance and support from ACLD.

Compensatory Instruction Guidelines

What does the term *compensatory instruction* mean in practical terms? All the suggestions listed below are based on the assumption that the key problem caused by perceptual skills dysfunction is a less-than-adequate ability to exploit what is already known in reading, spelling, and arithmetic—the basic coding systems of the classroom—in order to learn more; said more concisely, a poorly developed ability to associate new information with what is already known. This leads to an inability to remember enough of what is taught in any given instructional session, which then impairs associations and retention in subsequent instructional sessions, and so on. Admittedly, these statements represent a gross oversimplification of very complex processes, but that does not detract from their practical validity.

This reasoning implies that the child will be a more successful learner if the teacher does the following:

1. Make certain that the child really does have the factual information he will need to benefit from a given lesson. Assume nothing. Just because he seemed

to know something at an earlier time does not guarantee that he retains it. Find out.

2. Limit the amount of new information presented in any single lesson.

3. Make clear the system that links new information with the information the child already knows. (How *cat* links up with *hat;* how knowing 3 + 4 = 7 makes learning 4 + 3 = 7 significantly easier, etc.) The system should be made as explicit as is necessary and possible. Do not assume that the child will be able to figure it out on his own from what appear to be appropriate examples. Yes, he is likely to invent a system, but not an effective one. This happens all too frequently, meaning that the teacher then has to help the child unlearn some bad habits—behaviors established at an earlier time—before he can be taught proper ones.

4. Present new information in a way that highlights what is especially pertinent, what the child must pay special attention to if he is to learn from the lesson.

5. Try to teach the child how to generate his own mnemonics in those situations where basic systems do not apply.

6. Provide the child with enough repeated experiences (drill) to establish information securely in memory.

7. As the child practices and acquires a basic store of knowledge, show him how these can serve as "chunks"—larger units of analysis—in moving on to learning more complex units of information, for instance, recognizing such words as *scat,* and *scatter* because they contain the word *cat.*

8. Continue providing drill and practice as the concept of "chunking" is introduced and larger units of analysis are to be learned so that these, too, become part of the child's repertoire.

QUESTIONS AND ANSWERS ABOUT COMPENSATORY INSTRUCTION

The guidelines defined above often elicit questions from teachers and parents.

Q. What is the difference between a learning disability and dyslexia?

A. For all practical purposes, there is no difference between the two. At one time, dyslexia referred to a reading problem that was caused by specific damage to the central nervous system. Over time, the word has come to be used to describe all reading problems, regardless of cause.

Q. Shouldn't we find out if the child is a visual or auditory learner and then teach him accordingly?

A. No. This is a hard-to-put-to-rest idea; it sounds reasonable, but it does not work. In simple terms, the erroneous hypothesis is that some children have good visual analysis skills and poor auditory skills, or vice versa. Therefore, they should be taught to read with a sight (whole-word) method—a method that avoids explication of phonetic principles, or vice versa.

The fact is that learning to read cannot be reduced to modality preference constructs. Regardless of whether the child is deaf, blind, or has normal sight and hearing, reading is the process of mapping language onto symbols. With most children, therefore, it is the process of mapping oral language onto graphic symbols. To be able to do this, the child must be familiar with the oral language, the graphic symbols, and how the two are linked.

The 6-year-old child with appropriately developed auditory and visual perceptual skills will probably learn to read with any standard reading program, be it sight or phonics based or something in between. The same is true of the child with visual perceptual skills dysfunction, so long as his auditory analysis skills are adequate and his visual deficits are not so great as to impair his ability to learn to recognize the letters without confusion.

The child with auditory perceptual skills dysfunction, however, presents a different challenge. By definition, he lacks the ability to isolate the separate sounds (*phonemes* in the jargon of reading teachers) in the context of spoken words. Hence, he will not make satisfactory progress in a sight-reading program because it is not designed to make the separate phonemes apparent to him. He will not recognize the system; he certainly will not be able to memorize enough words by rote. He needs a reading program that *emphasizes* phonetic principles, a phonics program that makes clear to him what he cannot discover for himself because of his lack of auditory analysis skills.

Thus, the question is not, visual learner or auditory learner? Rather, it is, How important is it to teach the child phonetic principles with the child's TAAS score serving as the determinant.

Q. Where and how does spelling fit into this discussion? Is spelling affected by deficient visual or auditory perceptual skills? If so, which of the two is more important?

A. Spelling is affected by both abilities in different ways. The poor speller typically lacks one or both of the following: (1) the ability to analyze spoken words in terms of their phonemic elements, that is, auditory analysis skills; (2) the ability to invent mnemonics for remembering the correct letter sequences in those parts of words that are not spelled phonetically. Therefore, to help the poor speller, the teacher should attempt to improve the child's auditory analysis skills, if needed, and then teach the child useful mnemonics or inspire him to invent effective ones on his own.

A fundamental rule when teaching a mnemonic to a child is to keep it short and simple, and base it on something the child already knows well and can therefore build upon. Hence, there is no need to teach a mnemonic for remembering how to spell an entire word. Rather, teach a mnemonic for remembering that part of the word that is spelled irregularly—that is, non-phonetically, for example, "*i* before *e* except after *c*"; or have the child say the word to himself in a way that accentuates the spelling irregularity, for example, pronounce the /k/ sound in *knife* or the /h/ sound in *ghost*.

Q. How do these principles apply to helping a child who has difficulty with reading comprehension?

A. First of all, it is essential to make sure that the child understands the meaning of the words he is attempting to read and comprehend. If he is lacking in this, all other attempts at remediation will fail. Once this potential problem has been ruled out, consider his comprehension problem to be the product of poor organization skills. Show the child how to categorize information contained in stories and pictures, encouraging him to invent alternative organizations, and then to judge the relative effectiveness of each.

Q. Many children with substandard visual analysis skills also have poor handwriting. Will a child's handwriting improve if he is given visual analysis skills training?

A. Yes, handwriting is likely to improve as a result of visual analysis skills training. There are, however, faster, more direct ways of improving a child's handwriting; specifically, teach him the rules of penmanship, the mechanics that he did not learn when they were originally taught—if, indeed, they were taught. Teaching him those rules and having him practice them is bound to improve his handwriting. Simplistic? Yes. Effective? Absolutely.

Q. At what point should you worry about a child's tendency to reverse letters, for instance, to print the b for the *d?*

A. It is not uncommon for kindergarten-aged children and those even younger to reverse letters; hence, at that level, it is not cause for worry; however, there is no reason to allow even the young child to learn a bad habit if it can be avoided without difficulty. Hence, rather than worry, it is often helpful to teach the child a dependable mnemonic for distinguishing confusable letters, such as the *b* and *d*. One way to do this is to find a related letter that the child does not confuse—the capital *B*, perhaps. If he does not confuse its orientation, then it is but a small step to teach him that the lowercase *b* is "hidden" in the capital *B*. Refrain from the temptation to show how the *b* differs from the *d*. Ignore the *d*. Once the child has securely learned the *b*, the *d* will not present a problem; it will simply be the one that is not the *b*.

Q. Many schools provide bilingual programs for children who do not speak English upon entering school. Are the concepts discussed above applicable to them?

A. Yes. But one must keep in mind that the definition of reading is "mapping language onto symbols." If the child does not know the spoken language, he can hardly be expected to learn how to map it onto symbols. Such children are best served by first having time and experiences needed to learn the spoken language, then learning how to read it.

Q. Are these same concepts applicable to arithmetic?

A. Yes. Learning arithmetic is similar to learning to read in that the child has to learn to map language onto symbols. The difference is that there are two languages in arithmetic: a verbal one (the spoken words that pertain to arithmetic; e.g., *more, less, same as, one, two,* and *three*) and a nonverbal one (the recognition of such spatial attributes as quantity, magnitude, and relationship; in other words, visual analysis skills). The child should be familiar with both verbal and nonverbal languages when he begins formal instruction in arithmetic.

Factors the Patient Should Consider

Probable Outcome of Treatment. Assuming that prognosis is favorable, the child will display improved visual or auditory perceptual skills. As a result of this, he will also display the following:

If improvement occurs in visual analysis skills—*and if he is not already significantly behind in what he should know and be able to do in the classroom*—the child will demonstrate

a. Improved penmanship
b. Neater paperwork
c. A generally more organized approach to school activities
d. An improved ability to remember number facts: addition, subtraction, multiplication tables, etc.
e. An improved ability to invent effective mnemonic strategies, that is, systems that aid in the general ability to remember information.

If improvement occurs in auditory analysis skills—*and, again, if he is not already too far behind in school*—the child will also demonstrate

a. Improved word recognition skills, that is, he will recognize (read) words with increased speed and fluency
b. Improved capacity to associate new words with words he already knows; for example, knowing the word *ring* will facilitate his ability to read the words *ringing*, *bring*, *sing*, and *rang*.

Consequences If Recommendations Are Not Followed. A lack of compliance will probably result in a slow improvement in perceptual skills if the present condition is due to developmental lag rather than an organic or psychological factor but, along with this, a gradual and further deterioration of the child's classroom achievement (this is more fully discussed on pp. 107–108).

Patient's Obligations. The patient will be required to engage in about 30 minutes of prescribed remedial activities daily for approximately two to four months.

Number and Frequency of Office Visits. If all that is required is remediation of perceptual skills—that is, if there is no need for educational remediation—the patient should anticipate between three and six visits, depending on the level at which therapy begins and the rate at which he progresses. More specifically, if the patient begins therapy in either visual or auditory analysis skills at level I, anticipate four to six visits to complete the program, with about one month between each visit. If he begins in level II, anticipate three to four visits to complete the program, with about one month between each visit. If he begins in level III or higher, anticipate two to three visits to complete the program, with about one month between each visit.

Implementation of Therapy

Steps to be taken once the patient accepts the recommendation for remedial therapy.

1. Schedule Patient for a Second Visit. At that visit, the office assistant will carry out the sequence of procedures described in chapter 1 (pp. 1–4).

2. Placement Testing. Placement testing has already been done; it was accomplished when the screening tests were administered.

Tables 7.3 and 7.4 show how to translate the child's TVAS and TAAS scores into levels. For example, if the child TVAS score was zero, he placed in level I (Table 7.3); he has not mastered the visual analysis skills represented in the lowest level. If, instead, his score was 3, he would be in level III; he has mastered the lower two levels. Similarly, if his TAAS score was 3, he is placed in level III (Table 7.4); treatment can begin at this level.

3. Select Procedure. Select the appropriate procedure from Table 7.3 or 7.4. Locate it in the Procedures Manual, photocopy it, then follow the sequence described in chapter 1.

Perceptual skills therapy should be very straightforward. The main purpose is to emphasize analytic processes that teach the child, directly and clearly, how to get started in an auditory or visual analysis task in an efficient way, how to go to step 2 when step 1 has been accomplished, using what he accomplished at step 1 to help him complete step 2, what to do next, and so forth. It is neither a mystical nor a complex process. It does not require a recapitulation of all the developmental stages the child may have missed as he grew up.

4. Format of a Typical Follow-Up Visit

Obtain an updated history of the child's situation—what has been done at home, in school, and elsewhere since his last visit and what effects have been observed, for instance, has the assigned activity level been completed?

TABLE 7.3 TVAS Placement Table

TVAS Score	Place in level	Procedure
0	I	35, 43
1	II	36, 43
2–4	III	37, 43
5–8	IV	38
9–10	V	39
11–13	VI	40
14–15	VII	41
16–17	VIII	42

TABLE 7.4 TAAS Placement Table

TAAS Score	Place in level	Procedure
0	I	44, 50
1	II	45, 50
2–3	III	46, 50
4–6	IV	47
7–9	V	48
10–11	VI	49

Retest the child with the test or tests that initially identified his perceptual skills dysfunction: the TVAS or the TAAS. If the parent reported progress at home, it should be apparent in the child's performance on the test. If that, in fact, is the case, simply refer again to Table 7.3 or 7.4 to determine the child's present placement level and dispense the appropriate procedure(s). If, on the other hand, the child's in-office performance is not better than it was initially, a problem is indicated: either the parent is not following directions correctly or—worse yet—simply not following directions at all. In either event, the problem must be cleared up (see relevant suggestions on p. 5).

Determine what progress has been made in school. Typically, school progress lags behind improved perceptual skills, but if the prognostic guidelines defined above were followed (pp. 107–108), improved school performance should be apparent within a few months. If it is not, and if the patient's persistent classroom deficit is not due to the conditions spelled out in the discussion regarding factors that affect prognosis, then some reconsideration should be given to the possibility of an organic factor that might be impeding the child's progress. For example, the child's birth history may offer a clue that was initially overlooked. There is no need to terminate the therapy effort if that is the case, but there is a need to reconsider the prognosis in light of this potential stumbling block.

Continue with the postplacement testing sequence as defined on pp. 1–4.

CASE REPORTS

Patient 7.1

VISIT 1

Patient is a kindergarten student aged 5 years 10 months who was referred to us at the beginning of April, near the end of his kindergarten year.

Chief Complaints

Child's teacher has questioned the youngster's readiness for first grade. He has persistent difficulty completing simple paper-and-pencil tasks that do not challenge his classmates. In addition, he is not catching on to the letter-sound reading readiness lessons introduced a month or so ago—part of the regular curriculum in this middle-class neighborhood elementary school. Parents also observed that their son, their third and youngest child, has always been somewhat immature. Their question is, Does he have a perception problem, and should he enter first grade next year?

Child's health and developmental histories are uneventful: full-term delivery (Apgar = 9); no significant childhood diseases or trauma. He has never had an eye examination; neither has he ever manifested any related signs and symptoms.

Salient Clinical Data

Unaided visual acuity: 20/20 each eye

Ocular health: No evidence of pathology or structural abnormality

Refractive status: (OU) +0.50 D spheres

Binocular status

Stereoacuity

AT FAR	1 min of arc
AT NEAR	30 sec of arc

Cover test

AT FAR	Orthophoria
AT NEAR	5 PD exophoria

Binocular efficiency: Satisfactory vergence and accommodative facility

Perceptual skills

TVAS score = 2 (substandard for age)

TAAS score = 1 (substandard for age)

Parents are advised that child does not display an eye problem but does indeed show evidence of visual and auditory perceptual skills dysfunction. We recommend a program of remedial therapy to be administered by them at home. In respect to promotion to first grade, we defer to school and parent determination but also suggest that they put off any decision regarding this until after the child has engaged in therapy for a month or two. We also forewarn them that even if the therapy program proves to be successful—and we believe that prognosis is very favorable—their son might very well be served best by delaying entry into first grade until after his seventh birthday. (His June birthdate means that, if he does enter first grade next September, he will be among the youngest in the class—never a good idea for an immature child.)

Parents accept recommendation and schedule next visit.

VISIT 2 (ONE WEEK LATER)

Based upon TVAS and TAAS results obtained during the first visit, child is to commence this therapy on level III of the visual perceptual skills program and level II of the auditory skills program. As such, procedures 37, 38, 45, and 46 were photocopied, explained, and dispensed to the parent. (Because we usually schedule visits for these types of cases on a monthly basis, we dispensed both the level currently appropriate for the child and the level that follows it—this in anticipation that he may very well complete more than one level of perceptual skills activities within one month.)

When parents demonstrated understanding, an appointment was scheduled for a follow-up visit in one month. Parents were apprehensive about the long time between appointments; they were assured that they could always contact us if confusion or difficulty was encountered.

VISIT 3 (ONE MONTH LATER)

Parents report compliance and improvement; child has completed level III of the visual program and level II of the auditory. In addition, they report that his teacher is very pleased with his progress in school. He seems to have started to catch on, and the teacher is now inclined to think that he should enter first grade but acknowledges that he continues to lag behind his classmates.

Our assessment corroborates parents' reports:

TVAS score = 5

TAAS score = 3

This places the child in level IV of the visual program and level III of the auditory. Procedures 38 and 46 were given to the parents during their last visit; hence, only the two that follow them (39 and 47) are photocopied, explained to the parent, and dispensed. An appointment is scheduled for one month hence.

VISIT 4 (ONE MONTH LATER)

Parents report (and the daily log documents) compliance and improvement: child has completed level IV in the visual program and is making headway in level III of the auditory. School dismissed about two weeks ago. Child's teacher strongly urged parents to enroll him in first grade, attributing his sudden improvement to the fact that he is a late bloomer who caught up all of a sudden. We comment that the teacher might, indeed, be correct, but that it is just as likely that the child's gains are directly related to the parents' efforts at home to teach him the analysis skills he lacked and needs for elementary school. In any event, his gains are evident.

Retesting shows TVAS score = 8; TAAS score = 5 (but child appears to be uncertain in his responses to items 4 and 5).

Clearly, this is beyond what is usually shown by children just about to enter first grade. For all practical purposes, the remedial program may be stopped at this point. Child has mastered the skills he should have and has gone a bit beyond. There is no justification or benefit to be derived from additional treatment.

Parents are advised accordingly and asked to bring the child back to us for routine evaluation in about 8 to 12 months. We also advise them that, in our opinion, he is ready for the first grade but that this does not constitute a recommendation for entry into primary school at this time. He will be among the youngest in his class. That in itself is not a bad thing, but it could be. They should take this into consideration when they make their final decision about his placement in September.

Parents believe he would be better off in first grade because "he is tall for his age." We do not disagree.

VISIT 5 (SIX MONTHS LATER)

Child is in first grade and making satisfactory progress. He likes school, and his teacher has not observed anything to be concerned about.

Our examination, as well, reveals nothing of concern. His visual acuity, ocular health, refractive status, and binocular status are all well within normal limits. His perceptual skills remain a bit above what is expected from children at his grade level.

Parents are advised of our observations. Routine annual re-examination is recommended.

Patient 7.2

VISIT 1

Patient is a second-grade student aged 7 years 4 months who was referred to us in November. Parent's chief concern is that child is having trouble in school and teacher suspects "fine-motor-coordination problems and a short attention span." Parents say this refers to the fact that his pencil-and-paper work is "messy," that he does not seem to be able to follow directions or figure out for himself how to get through anything but the simplest of tasks, and that, in general, he is "disorganized." They also inform us that his birth, development, and health histories are uneventful. He experienced no difficulties in kindergarten or first grade. They did observe, however, that his first-grade paperwork was rather sloppy but that his teacher that year did not seem to be very concerned about it. Further questioning revealed that his first-grade teacher was a very "loving" lady who referred to the students as "her babies" and was inclined to think that school performance difficulties would be "grown out of."

Salient Clinical Data

Unaided visual acuity: 20/20 each eye

Ocular health: No evidence of pathology or structural abnormality

Refractive status: (OU) +0.75 −0.25 cx 180

Binocular status

Stereoacuity
AT FAR 1 min of arc
AT NEAR 40 sec of arc

Cover test
AT FAR 1 PD esophoria
AT NEAR 3 PD exophoria

Binocular efficiency: Satisfactory vergence and accommodative facility

Perceptual skills

TVAS score = 6 (substandard for age)
TAAS score = 9 (appropriate for age)

Parents are advised that child's classroom problems do not stem from a need for glasses or poor binocular coordination. His visual perceptual skills, however, are lagging; his auditory skills, in contrast, are at a satisfactory level for his grade. We also note that this matches up with his classroom record. He is progressing appropriately in reading; something his TAAS score would suggest. He is not progressing appropriately in activities that link closely with spatial organization abilities, and this is corroborated by his less-than-adequate TVAS score.

We recommend a program of remedial therapy to be administered at home. We also suggest that while this is going on the child's teacher be asked to modify her instructional approach with the child in ways that take into account his general lack of organization; that she provide him the structure that he cannot supply for himself. As examples, we urge that when he is to complete a paper-and-pencil activity he be told in unambiguous terms what to do first, what to do next, and so on; what to pay particular attention to and why. We also stress that the teacher be reassured that this is not a long-term need. Prognosis is very favorable. The child is not yet very far behind in school, his motivation appears to be excellent, and his parents are obviously committed to helping him overcome his problems. Hence, one can be more or less optimistic about predicting that if the therapy program is complied with, reasonable improvement in school can be expected within three to five months.

Parents accept recommendation and schedule the next visit, at which time they will be given directions for the remedial therapy program.

VISIT 2 (ONE WEEK LATER)

On the basis of the child's TVAS score obtained during the first visit, child is to commence this therapy on level IV. Procedures 38 and 39 were photocopied and explained to the parent. (As with patient 7.1, we dispensed the level appropriate for the child and the level that follows it in anticipation that the child might complete more than one level of perceptual skills activities before the next visit.)

When parents demonstrated understanding, child was given an appointment for a follow-up visit one month hence.

VISIT 3 (ONE MONTH LATER)

Parents report improvement; child has completed level IV in the visual program and is about halfway through level V. In addition, they report that he might be making some improvement in school. According to his teacher, he continues to be inattentive and unable to work independently on anything except the simplest of tasks, but what he does complete now "looks better, neater, better organized." This pleases the teacher and the parents. Indeed, it pleases us as well in that these observations are often noted after about a month of therapy in those cases where the final outcomes are excellent.

Our assessment agrees with parent's reports; TVAS score = 9.

This places the child in level V of the visual program—just where he is. Parents are therefore advised to continue as is and are given the activities for level VI as well (procedure 40), these to be implemented when and if the child completes the level he is now working on. An appointment is scheduled for one month hence.

VISIT 4 (ONE MONTH LATER)

Parents report compliance and significant school improvement; they have been advised that the child is much less dependent upon his teacher for directions and guidance in completing desk activities. Indeed, his attention span has improved and, for that matter, so has his arithmetic achievement—something that had not really concerned his teacher in the past, but that is pleasing nonetheless. In the teacher's words, he has "gotten into gear." Parents also reported progress in the therapy program. Child completed level V during the past month. He seems to be making steady progress and is now able to work through the activities at a reasonable rate.

Retesting shows TVAS score = 11; this places the child in level VI. Parents are given the activities for level VII (procedure 41)—they already have the activities for level VI—and asked to return in one month.

VISIT 5 (ONE MONTH LATER)

Parents report continued improvement. Child's teacher believes that he is cured. His day-to-day classroom work is, at the least, satisfactory, and sometimes it surpasses that level. He is now able to complete work as independently as any of the children in his class. The teacher is pleased about results, and particularly pleased about having been the one who identified the difficulty and made the referral. Obviously, parents are also very pleased. In respect to his therapy, parents state that child completed level VI during the past month and has not worked as hard as before on level VII. They also acknowledge that they are not as motivated as before; his excellent improvement in school has made them comfortable.

Retesting shows TVAS score = 14; this places the child in level VII, the level he is currently working in. Parents are advised to try to complete that level during the next month, then to cease the therapy. We inform them that they need not return to this office for about four months unless something unforeseen or troublesome arises in the interim. Our prediction is that the child will perform satisfactorily in school, although we also assure them that he is human, after all, and will undoubtedly have days when things do not go right.

VISIT 6 (FOUR MONTHS LATER)

Parents report no problems. Child is progressing satisfactorily in school. Our reassessment confirms their comments. TVAS score = 16. Cursory reassessment of his ocular status reveals no changes from initial visit. Parents are reassured and advised to return in one year for routine reexamination.

Patient 7.3

VISIT 1

Patient is a 10-year-old, fourth-grade student who was referred to us because of learning difficulties.

Chief Complaints

He has had trouble in school since first grade, especially in reading. Third-grade achievement tests show him to be reading at an end-of-first-grade level; achievement in spelling is also well behind; he scored satisfactorily in other subject areas. He has had previous eye examinations; no problems have ever been identified. He has also had psychological evaluation; his IQ is within normal limits. His birth and developmental histories are uneventful with the exception of a very slight delay in language development. His health has been good, although here, too, there is one exception: he has been subject to recurring ear infections and has had drainage tubes inserted on two occasions, once at age 3, again about a year later. His hearing, tested a few months ago, is normal. His teacher has had considerable experience in tutoring problem readers but has not yet made much headway with this child and believes that his main problem is substandard word-recognition (or decoding) skills; that is, he has great trouble remembering what the printed words say and often resorts to guessing—sometimes without any apparent system, sometimes by enunciating the sound of the first letter of a word and guessing at the rest. The teacher believes that the child is a "nice boy," motivated and polite, but has expressed concern lately that he may be less motivated than he used to be, attributing this to discouragement: he has tried to do better in school but has not been successful.

Salient Clinical Data

Unaided visual acuity: 20/20 each eye

Ocular health: No evidence of pathology or structural abnormality

Refractive status: (OU) +050 −0.50 cx 180

Binocular status

Stereoacuity

AT FAR	1 min of arc
AT NEAR	20 sec of arc

Cover test

AT FAR	Orthophoria
AT NEAR	5 PD exophoria

Binocular efficiency: Satisfactory vergence and accommodative facility

Perceptual skills

TVAS score = 16 (appropriate for grade)
TAAS score = 8 (substandard for grade)

Parents are advised that child's classroom problems do not stem from a need for glasses or any other eye problem. His visual perceptual skills appear to be properly developed. The only deficit we noted was substandard auditory analysis skills. This is not surprising, however, in that auditory analysis skills and word-recognition skills have often been shown to be closely correlated.

Treatment options were discussed with the parents. It would appear on the surface that the best option would be remediation to improve the child's auditory analysis skills. That is not correct reasoning, however. True enough, his auditory analysis skills are deficient; also true is that this deficiency probably has contributed mightily to his inadequate word-recognition skills, which, in turn, must be impeding his general reading achievement. But it also must be kept in mind that he is in fourth grade and functioning about three years behind in reading. Improving his auditory analysis skills will not improve his reading; he will continue to lag. Improved auditory analysis skills will simply improve his aptitude for learning to read. Someone will still have to teach him, and the task will not be easy considering his age, grade, and present reading ability.

We therefore recommend that a report be forwarded to the child's school. Contained in that report should be (1) documentation of his auditory perceptual skills deficit; (2) a strong recommendation that the child be provided with additional help in those aspects of this schooling where help is needed, specifically, that he be taught reading and spelling in ways that accommodate his substandard auditory analysis skills; and (3) a recommendation that perceptual skills remediation be provided as part of the child's regular school day.

Parents agree. Report is written. School subsequently contacts us to seek more specific information regarding (1) what the perceptual skills remediation program comprises, and (2) the nature of the special classroom help that would best aid this child.

We respond by providing them with the auditory analysis skills procedures (44–50), the compensatory instruction guidelines defined on pp. 110–111, and some general discussion regarding the problem. We also offer to monitor the child's progress on a monthly basis and collaborate with them as indicated.

School and parents agree to this arrangement.

VISIT 6 (18 MONTHS LATER)

We have seen this patient four times since his first visit. He has made excellent progress. His auditory analysis skills have improved remarkably; so has his reading. The first can be attributed to the fact that his teacher supervised the skills training program very conscientiously. The second, to fact that in addition to improving the child's auditory analysis skills, his teacher modified reading instruction to stress phonic principles and then showed the child how a good reader, once he has learned some basic reading skills, "chunks" single letters and their respective sounds into strings of letters that typically have the same sound regardless of the word in which they occur; for example, not only does the letter *k* have a /k/ sound, but the letter string *ake* is almost always pronounced as it is in the word *cake; ing* as in *sing,* and so on.

Parents are very grateful. School anticipates placing him in a regular program at the end of this school year; he is overcoming his academic lag.

Not all case reports end on such happy notes. We cannot stress too much the importance of appropriate instructional conditions, particularly for children who are in fourth grade and higher. As already noted, with older children it is not simply a question of improving perceptual skills; if they are to make satisfactory progress in school, their educational lag also has to be overcome.

CHAPTER 8

Management

This chapter addresses the following topics:

1. The office assistant—his or her role and how to prepare for it
2. Instruments. What and how many are needed; their functions—what they do and how they do it; their critical similarities and differences; where to procure them and at what cost; how to produce certain devices in your own office; different ways to distribute instruments to patients for home use.
3. Effective use of office space
4. Fees

THE OFFICE ASSISTANT

The pivotal individual in providing vision therapy in a primary-care optometric practice is a competent, knowledgeable office assistant. Without such a person, cost-effective management of vision therapy is hardly possible. Thus, the question arises, where does the optometrist seek such an individual? Unfortunately, it is not simply a matter of contacting a school and requesting names of its graduates. There are very few, if any, formal educational programs. Hence, the best (and perhaps only) solution is for the optometrist to provide the training program.

The first step is to identify an individual who exhibits the traits required for such a position. Although the following list is not all-inclusive, it is reasonable to suggest that the office assistant be

1. Intelligent—able to interpret the directions described in the procedures, and the observations and reactions provided by the patients.

2. Patient—willing to explain a procedure slowly and carefully, then to re-explain it if necessary.

3. Articulate—able to communicate effectively with the patients and optometrist.

4. Intellectually curious and motivated; interested in learning new skills and information.

5. Compassionate—able to provide encouragement when the patient's enthusiasm starts to wane because of a slowdown in progress.

6. Binocular—the office assistant who lacks adequate binocularity will probably not be able to comprehend fully just what it is that the patient should be able to do in therapy procedures that involve binocular functions. As such, his or her effectiveness as a manager of those treatment programs is apt to be impaired. This is unfortunate, but it is a fact. The office assistant who is not able to perceive what the patient is attempting to learn—although intelligent, patient, articulate, compassionate, intellectually curious, and motivated—will probably fall short when it comes to providing the kind of information and guidance patients need in order to benefit from vision therapy.

Sources of Information

There is not a great deal of printed material available, but the following will be helpful:

1. The papers published over the years by the Optometric Extension Program, Duncan, Oklahoma, for office assistants. These contain much information, some of which is directly relevant. Unfortunately, a good deal of scanning will be needed to identify those segments that are most useful.

2. Books and journals related to orthoptics, child development, perceptual skills development as it pertains to school achievement, etc. (See Bibliography for some suggestions.)

Other experiences that would be helpful:

1. Encourage and arrange for the office assistant to visit the offices of colleagues who have already trained their assistants to manage vision therapy programs.

2. Have the assistant read this book and, most important, work through all of the procedures, step by step, as though he or she were a patient.

3. Encourage the assistant to attend continuing education courses that address these topics and are designed for his or her level of knowledge.

4. Explain to the assistant, in lay terms, the clinical conditions and treatments discussed in this book. The assistant's goal is to learn how to do this same thing for patients. To this end, included below are explanations of the various conditions,

written in language that the average adult will be able to understand. The assistant should become familiar with these, use them with patients, and in time—as the information becomes more familiar and better understood—enrich them with personalized variations.

Vergence Infacility Inefficient binocular (two-eyed) coordination; i.e., the patient uses his two eyes together, but not in a facile manner. Hence, despite good eyesight (with or without glasses), he often experiences discomfort symptoms (e.g., headaches or fatigue), especially when reading or doing other close work. The following explanation usually satisfies the average patient:

> There are two sets of eye muscles involved in vision. One set may be called the "aiming" or "pointing" [vergence] muscles; these control where the eyes are fixating—for example, to the left, up, down, to the right, or up close. The other set may be referred to as the "focusing" [accommodation] muscles. These provide the *extra* focusing power the eyes need to see something clearly when it is held close. [The normal eye has enough built-in optical power to see clearly at distance without calling upon the focusing muscles.] In a way, it is analogous to using a pair of magnifying binoculars; you must point them and focus. [It is the focusing muscles that typically weaken when a person approaches age 40, thereby necessitating the use of reading glasses or bifocals.]
>
> The two sets of muscles—pointing and focusing—work together. When normal eyes look at something far away—that is, across a room or even further—the focusing muscles automatically relax as the pointing muscles maintain the eyes in straight-ahead position. Then, when these same normal eyes look at something up close, such as a printed page, the pointing muscles turn the eyes inward (converge) toward the nose, and at the same time (again, automatically), the focusing muscles go to work to provide the extra power needed, because it is close, to see the print clearly. These two actions are linked together as a reflex; when either set goes into action—the pointing muscles or the focusing muscles—the other does likewise, automatically. Similarly, when either set relaxes, so does the other.
>
> This link between the pointing and focusing muscles should not be too tight; there should be some flexibility between the two—each should be able to be exercised or relaxed to some degree without having an equal effect on the other. Consider an comparable situation: Most of us can stand erect on level ground. Most of us can also stand erect on a slope or while balancing some weight on one shoulder. We do this by adjusting the interrelationships of the various body parts that participate in our maintaining an upright posture. It is good that we can do this; it indicates an adaptability that is essential to efficient posture; it means we can shift our weight with sufficient ease to ward off strain. If we could stand erect only on level ground and fell over when attempting to do this on a slope or while balancing a weight on one shoulder, it would suggest a less-than-satisfactory ability to adapt, to reorganize the postural mechanisms of the body in a way that indicates efficient body management.
>
> The same principles apply to vision. A certain amount of slack—adaptability—between the pointing and focusing systems of the eyes is a good thing. Some

patients lack it. If that lacking appears to be in the pointing muscles, it is called vergence infacility.

Treatment of vergence infacility involves teaching the patient how to use (activate and relax) his pointing muscles somewhat independent of his focusing muscles.

Accommodation Infacility. Inefficient binocular (two-eyed) coordination that greatly resembles vergence infacility except that the lack of adaptability is in the focusing (accommodating) muscles rather than in the pointing muscles. Hence, its treatment typically involves teaching the patient how to use (activate and relax) his focusing muscles somewhat independent of his pointing muscles.

Binocular Instability. This refers to a condition where the patient's eyes are in alignment (straight) some of the time, and out-of-alignment (crossed or turned out) at other times. It frequently occurs as *intermittent strabismus;* "strabismus" refers to eyes that are not in correct alignment; "intermittent" indicates that the condition is not constant—it occurs from time to time. Binocular instability may be caused by weak eye (pointing) muscles or by damaged nerves. In the majority of cases, however, it is due to poor binocular coordination—the two eyes do not consistently work together as efficiently (quickly and accurately) as they should, despite the fact that the eye muscles and nerves are perfectly normal. Its treatment, therefore, involves teaching the patient how to coordinate his two eyes with accuracy and ease.

Convergence Insufficiency. A condition of binocular instability in which the patient has difficulty keeping both eyes fixed (converged) on a near target; e.g., directed at a target that is held any closer than 9 in or so from his eyes. This is not ordinarily caused by weak eye muscles; it is a binocular coordination problem.

To illustrate this point, have the patient look at a near-point object with one eye or look at himself in a mirror. (The other eye is to be covered.) Move the fixation object closer to the patient, or have the patient rotate his head as he continues to look in the mirror, so that his uncovered eye is turned in (converged) as far toward his nose as possible. Both of these circumstances will demonstrate to the patient that this eye, at least, is able to turn all the way in. Then move the occluder to the other eye, have the patient fixate the object (or, again, look into the mirror) with the eye that was initially covered and repeat the activity, demonstrating to the patient that this eye, as well, is capable of turning all the way in.

Now uncover both eyes and have the patient fixate an object as it is moved closer to his nose. If he does, in fact, have a convergence insufficiency, he will be unable to converge both eyes to the extent that he could when fixating with one eye only. The explanation for this is not weak muscles, obviously; each eye turned in toward the nose with relatively little difficulty when it operated independent of the partner eye. The only other plausible cause is poor binocular coordination.

Accommodative Esotropia. A condition of binocular instability wherein one eye crosses (turns inward—toward the nose—more than it should) when the patient uses his focusing muscles to see an object clearly. This is most likely to occur in certain farsighted (*hyperopic*) persons when they are not wearing their glasses. It may also occur even when they are wearing their glasses and looking at a near object, that is, one located within arm's range. (This latter condition is called *convergence excess.*) Once again, this cannot be attributed to weak or extra strong eye muscles; it is a problem in binocular coordination, but a bit more difficult to explain than convergence insufficiency.

The following, when combined with the discussion about vergence infacility, usually explains it adequately:

> Farsighted eyes are not as strong as they should be in basic optical—focusing—power. That is what earns them the label *farsighted.* Therefore, when the farsighted patient looks at something far away, he will not see clearly unless his focusing muscles go to work to provide extra power—power that his eyes lack because of the farsightedness. When the focusing muscles do this, the brain sends a reflex-driven [automatic] signal to the pointing muscles that, in turn, causes them to turn the eyes inward. This is why some farsighted children become cross-eyed when they are 18 to 24 months old and continue to be cross-eyed when they remove their glasses.
>
> In some people, both farsighted and not farsighted, the reflex hookup between the pointing and focusing muscles is not properly synchronized. Their pointing muscles overreact to signals from their focusing muscles whether they are wearing their glasses or not. Therefore, when they look at something up close, necessitating that their focusing muscles to go to work, the signal to the pointing muscles is too strong, and one eye turns in too much.

In both of these conditions, vision therapy can be very helpful, but more often than not, glasses—sometimes single vision, sometimes bifocal—are also needed.

Divergence Excess. A condition in which one eye turns out when the patient is staring off into distance; most often, when he is fatigued or not looking at something specific but merely gazing in a daydreamlike way.

The following, when combined with the basic information about the pointing and focusing muscles presented in the discussion of vergence infacility, usually explains this condition adequately to the patient:

> There is a direct reflex link between the pointing and focusing muscles of the eyes. For some reason or other, not known at present, some patients' pointing muscles overrelax when their focusing muscles relax.
>
> Staring off into the distance causes the focusing muscles to relax; this, in turn, causes the pointing muscles to overrelax, and one eye turns out, at least until the patient snaps out of his stare and starts to look at [focus on] things more precisely. Then the eyes come into normal alignment.

The goal of vision therapy in this type of case is to train the pointing muscles to not overrelax when the eyes are directed to distance.

Amblyopia. The normal newborn child does not see very clearly. But if his visual system (eyes and the nerves that support them) are normal, and if nothing occurs to alter that state, he will develop clear eyesight within the first three or four years of life, with the most dramatic improvement occurring during the first year or so.

Unfortunately, some children are not born with a normal visual system—for example, one or both of their eyes may be very hyperopic (farsighted) or astigmatic; he may be *strabismic* (one eye out of line) or have a *cataract* (the lens in the eye is not completely transparent); or he may have a *ptosis* (an eyelid that droops) to the extent that it obstructs sight. When an eye—albeit normal at birth—does not experience unobstructed, focused vision during the first few years of life, it becomes *amblyopic* (lazy), that is, unable to see clearly even if, subsequently, the necessary lenses are supplied or the obstruction is removed. In effect, it is similar to what would happen to an arm or a leg that was kept immobilized for the first few years of life. Normal development is hampered and the effects are lifelong.

When treatment is feasible—as determined by the optometrist—it usually involves forcing the amblyopic eye to work under controlled conditions; sometimes necessitating a patch over the good eye, sometimes involving the use of binocular equipment of one sort or another (see, for example, procedures 28–34).

Visual Perceptual (Analysis) Skills Dysfunction. A condition wherein the child is not as aware as he should be (considering his age or grade) of certain important details in what he is looking at. He reveals this in his responses to such tests as the TVAS, as well as in how he completes paper-and-pencil activities in school (see chapter 7 for a fuller description of this). The following usually explains this condition to a parent's or teacher's satisfaction:

> It might seem reasonable to attribute the child's inadequate responses to the TVAS or any other copying tests to substandard fine motor skills. But that is very rarely the correct explanation. [See suggestions for illustrating this on p. 103.] It probably also seems reasonable to speculate that the child's difficulties are caused by the fact that he literally sees things in a distorted manner. For all practical purposes, this is never the case. [See suggestions for illustrating this on p. 102.]
>
> The best way to understand the child's responses to these tests is for you, yourself, to try to draw, with complete accuracy, something that is full of details: a tree in full leaf, for example, or the randomly perforated acoustical tiles that serve as ceilings in many offices. Seeing something clearly hardly means you will be able to reproduce it accurately. The latter requires a very precise, detailed, step-by-step analysis of what you are looking at and trying to draw, far more precise than when you are merely identifying it.
>
> [It sometimes is useful to have the parent attempt to perform such a task, just to reinforce the great difference between seeing something clearly and being able to analyze it to the level where it can be reproduced.]
>
> The child with a visual perceptual skills problem is not demonstrating a sight problem; he has an analysis problem, just as you do when you try to copy a tree in full leaf. But there is a crucial difference in his situation. The task we just proposed for you, the adult, would be too difficult for any adult. Just about everyone would encounter the same difficulties. The child with visual perceptual skills dysfunction does not have that much company; his problem is not so wide-

spread; most of his classmates do not encounter the difficulty he does in analyzing concrete information. Hence, his teacher, in a standard classroom, will use lessons and instructional materials that presume this fundamental analysis ability and not be disappointed by most of the children in the class, only by those with visual perceptual skills deficits. That group will fail to learn adequately in those lessons where visual perceptual skills are needed. This, repeated over days and months, culminates in a significant lag in classroom learning, which, in itself—independent of the visual perceptual skills deficit—will significantly compound the child's learning problems.

Treatment of visual perceptual skills, therefore, involves teaching the child how to go about analyzing spatial information in an organized way—that is, breaking it down into its separate parts—and recognizing, or mapping out, the relationships among those parts in a systematic, step-by-step manner. We start off by teaching him, with geometric designs, that he *must first* identify a single component, *then* another, *then* another. We also teach him how to read a simple map—pins on a geoboard and related dots arranged within the boundaries of a printed square. As the child progresses, we will increase the complexity of the patterns he is to analyze in terms of their components and the map he uses for representing relationships. Eventually, and only as the child shows the ability to move on, we will teach him how to map out relationships even when most of the mapping cues are removed; in general terms, he will be taught how to use the information that is available to good advantage.

As he achieves these goals, the first- or second-grade child will demonstrate what he has learned by being more organized in his paperwork, his ability to remember information regardless of how it is received—through the eyes or the ears, his performance in arithmetic, and his reading comprehension skills. With older children, the effects will not be so apparent *if* the child is also lagging significantly in his schoolwork. Improving his visual perceptual skills only makes him better prepared to learn in a standard classroom; it does not teach him the information he failed to learn because he entered school with inadequate visual perceptual skills—it is a little like starting to run for a train after it has left the station. Hence, improved visual perceptual skills is only part of his aims; he also needs good remedial instruction.

Auditory Perceptual (Analysis) Skills Dysfunction. A condition wherein the child is not as aware of acoustical details as he should be, considering his age or grade. More specifically, a condition wherein the child is not as aware of the separate sounds in spoken words as other children of the same age or grade.

The illustrating explanations of this condition are similar to what was offered above in respect to visual analysis skills deficits. The only real difference is that with this condition there is lack of awareness of acoustical details rather than visual ones. Just as with the analysis of visual details, children become more adept at analyzing acoustical information through growth and development. One of the things they learn is that spoken words not only have meaning but also consist of sounds arranged in specific sequences; as such, they have lots of discrete similarities and differences in the sounds they do and do not contain. As children gain this awareness, they start to recognize the cogent and related (similar or different) characteristics in such spoken words as *say*, *may*, *day* and *date*.

Children who lack these abilities perplex their teachers: most of the children in a typical first-grade class are able to remember what the printed words in their books say; these few cannot. True, even the more adept students in the class will forget a word from time to time. But they will have a good method for then recalling that word, usually by associating some of the details of the printed word they are trying to identify with related similarities and differences in other words that they do remember, thereby triggering recognition of the word they were after; for example, if they forget what *pit* says but remember *sit* and *fit* and are cognizant of the acoustical similarities and differences of these three words as well as the visual, then they are very likely to remember what *pit* says after a second or two of thinking (i.e., searching memory in an organized way).

Treatment, therefore, involves teaching the child how to go about analyzing spoken words in terms of their separate parts (sounds) and recognizing (mapping out) the relationships among those parts in a systematic, step-by-step manner. This is begun by (if the child needs to start at such a basic level) teaching him how to break a spoken two-syllable compound word (e.g., *cupcake*) into its separate syllables; then, how to do the same with polysyllabic words in which the syllables are not meaningful (e.g., *vacation*). Then the focus is shifted to single sounds, first those that start a word, then final sounds, then sounds that are part of a consonant blend, for instance, the /t/ sound in the word *track*.

As these goals are achieved, the first- or second-grade child will demonstrate what he has learned by improved performance in reading and, to some extent, spelling. With older children, the effects will not be so apparent *if* the child is also lagging significantly in his schoolwork. Improving his auditory perceptual skills only makes him better prepared to learn certain things in a standard classroom; it does not teach him the information he failed to learn because he entered school with inadequate auditory perceptual skills. Hence, improved auditory perceptual skill is only part of his aims; he also needs good remedial instruction.

INSTRUMENTS

There is no need, at the onset, to purchase a large inventory of equipment. Obviously, the number of any given device that is kept on hand can be modified at any time in accord with the optometrist's or assistant's individual preferences. A suggested start-up inventory is listed in Table 8.1; each of these items is then described in a way that the optometrist will certainly comprehend but that the assistant may not—at least at first. To understand these devices, the assistant should, first, read the information below, taking from it what he or she can and asking the optometrist to clear up confusing points; then he or she should work through the procedures in the procedures manual, trying to relate what is done as they engage in the therapy activities to what has been read; then the assistant should re-read the information below. It will make better sense the second time through. (Note to assistant: When vergence is referred to below, think of it as the action of the pointing muscles; when accommodation

TABLE 8.1 Basic Instrument Inventory

Instrument	Catalog no.	Cost[b]	Source[c]
Aperture Rule	BC/1050	$ 25.00	1
Variable-Mirror Stereoscope	BC/405MSE	58.00	1
SOMS Trainer (single-mirror stereoscope)	BC/160	75.00	1
Horizontal minivectograms kit[a]	BC/275MVH	24.00	1
Vertical minivectograms kit	BC/216MVK	25.00	1
Minitranaglyphs	BC/920	11.00	1
Hand-held Biopter (Brewster stereoscope)	SO/N-108	55.00	1
Prism Base-Out Story Book Cards	BC/BO-A	6.00	1
Prism Base-In Story Book Cards	BC/BI-A	6.00	1
Red-Green TV Trainer	BC/63RG	18.00	1
Red-Green Stereo Trainer	BC906	11.50	1
Quoit vectograms	SO/V2	55.00	1
Vectogram 9 (nonvariable)	SO/V9	20.00	1
Lens holder (4-cell)	BC/LH4	14.00	1
Square plastic prisms			
0.5–10 D	G/SP-37A	6.00	1
12–20 D	G/SP-37B	6.00	1
25–35 D	G/SP-37C	7.00	1
40–50 D	G/SP-37D	7.00	1
Horizontal prism bar			
6 powers: 1–20 D	G/B-6	40.00	1
16 powers: 1–45 D	G/B-15	75.00	1
Vertical prism bar			
10 powers: 0.5–10 D	G/B-10	55.00	1
Phy-Dip Trainer	BC/1091	4.00	1
Red-Green Tranaglyph Kit (5 sets variable tranaglyphs)	BC/600K	45.00	1
Red-Green Tranaglyph Kit (6 nonvariable tranaglyphs)	BC/50K	29.00	1
Polarizing goggles (pkg of 6)	BC/PG	30.00	1
Red-Green goggles (pkg of 6)	BC/1180	19.00	1
Red-Green bar reader	BC/1316	4.00	1
Red-Green Stereo Trainer	BC/906	11.50	1
Keystone (Brewster) stereoscope[a]	725–030	54.00	2
Children's stories, base-out	005–154	30.00	2
Children's stories, base-in	005–153	30.00	2
Adult Comfort Kit, base-out	005–151	30.00	2
Keystone (Brewster) cheiroscope[a]	725–000	225.00	2

[a] These instruments may be omitted from a start-up inventory and added latter, as needed or wanted.
[b] From manufacturer's 1986 catalog.
[c] 1 = Bernell Manufacturing Co.; 750 Lincolnway East (P.O. Box 4637); South Bend, IN 46634
2 = Keystone View; Mast Development Company; 2212 East 12th Street; Davenport, IA 52803

is mentioned, think of that as the action of the focusing muscles. See pp. 126–127 for additional information regarding this.)

Although they differ in how they function, most of the instruments listed in Table 8.1 that are designed for improving binocular efficiency serve the same general purpose: they provide the patient with the conditions for learning how to activate or inhibit vergence independent of accommodation, or vice versa. In other words, they all have the capacity—even further enhanced when used in conjunction with plus and minus spherical lenses—to teach the patient how to converge or diverge (i.e., how to adjust his pointing muscles) while accommodating, holding accommodation constant, or relaxing accommodation (i.e., doing something different with his focusing muscles). The goal is not to make the one function totally independent of the other but, rather, to teach the patient how to use his visual system more efficiently—with greater adaptability.

Aperture Rule. This instrument (see Figure 8.1) allows for stimulating fusional convergence or divergence independent of accommodation by presenting separate targets to each eye that can be fused (merged) into a single image only when the patient fixates at the correct point in space, and seen clearly, at the same time, only if the patient accommodates for a different location in space.

The key feature of this device is the so-called aperture slide. There are two of these. One has a single aperture (vertical rectangular slot) in the middle of it; the other (double aperture) slide has two rectangular slots. Also supplied with the instrument is a booklet of pairs of targets, each designated by a number that indicates in centimeters the center-to-center separation between the pairs of targets (AP1 targets are 1 cm apart, center-to-center, AP2 targets are 2 cm apart, and so on.)*

The targets are positioned on the rule in such a way that when an aperture slide (either one) is in its proper place, the patient will be able to see only one target with one eye, and the other target with the other eye, even when both eyes are open. (If a base-out demand is wanted, the targets should be in a *cross-disparity condition*—that is, the right target is visible to the patient's left eye and vice versa—this calls for the single-aperture slide. If a base-in demand is wanted, the targets should be in an *uncrossed-disparity condition*—that is, the right target is visible to the right eye, and the left target to the left eye—this calls for the double-aperture slide.) The patient's job is to fuse the pair of targets into a single image and to keep that image clear. As noted above, he accomplishes this by learning how to converge to one point in space while accommodating for another location.

If the single-aperture slide is used, the patient will have to exercise positive vergence (converge) in excess of accommodation to fuse the targets into a single, clear image. (This is also called *chiastopic fusion.*) In other words, the patient will have to fixate in front of where the targets are actually positioned; specifically, at the plane of the aperture. At the same time, he will have to keep accommodation fixed on the plane of the actual targets in order to maintain clarity. Because the targets are farther away from the patient than is the aperture slide, this requires positive relative convergence. The patient will sense this as forcing him to work harder to fuse the images. He should be encouraged in this regard.

If the double-aperture slide is used, the reverse situation is produced. The patient has to inhibit vergence (diverge) in relation to accommodation in order to fuse the targets into a single and clear image. (This is also called *orthopic* fusion). The patient will sense this as requiring him to relax as he tries to fuse the images. Most patients

* The formula for calculating the fusional demand in prism diopters is

$$\text{PD} = \frac{\text{separation of targets (cm)}}{\text{viewing distance (m)}}$$

Hence, when viewed from a distance of 1 m, targets separated by 1 cm will represent a fusion demand of 1 PD, when these same targets are viewed from a distance of 0.5 m, they will represent a demand of 2 PD, etc.

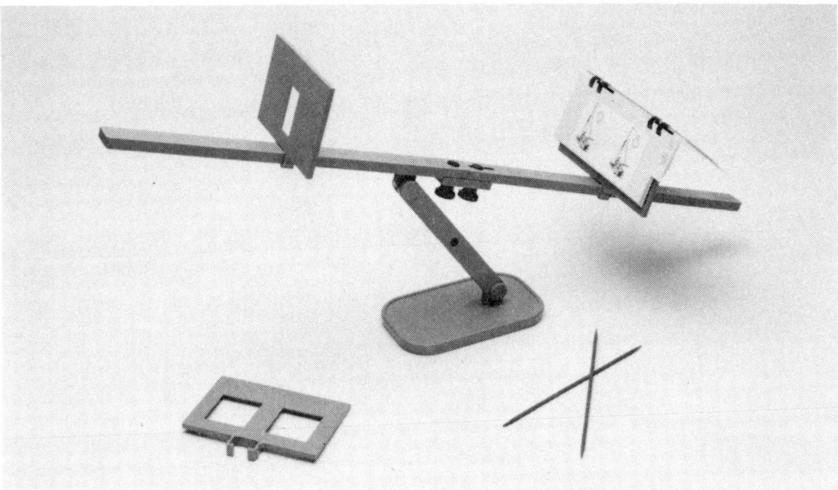

FIGURE 8.1 Aperture Rule

find divergence more difficult than convergence. But if that is what is to be learned, then so be it. It certainly can be accomplished. As such, it is often helpful when working on negative relative convergence ranges (base-in demand) to have the patient engage in the prescribed activities while seated comfortably in a chair that allows him to settle back, hold the aperture rule in his hand in a way that requires him to elevate his gaze, and relax, allowing the two targets to float together.

The aperture rule may also be used without an aperture slide (see procedure 2). Under those conditions, fusing the two targets will cause the patient to see three images. In other words, if he fixates at the correct point (as if an aperture slide [either] were in place), he will see a fused image (a composite of what the right eye and left eye sees), and he will see the two additional targets as well (one belonging to the right eye, the other to the left). These latter are not visible to the patient when an aperture slide (either) is used. Hence, this procedure is more difficult in that the patient has to ignore the distracting extra images. On the other hand, it is a useful procedure for bridging the gap between the basic aperture rule procedure (procedure 1) and the chiastopic and orthopic (instrument-free) fusion techniques called for in the three parts of procedure 3. The main advantage of procedure 2 over procedure 3 is that in the former the rule provides the patient with a way of determining where to fixate in order to obtain fusion. This is a very useful aid in moving from instrument-controlled activities to those that are instrument-free.

Stereoscope. There are two different kinds of stereoscopes, but in practical terms, they function more or less the same. Both types, like the aperture rule described above, are designed to present to each eye a different target that the patient learns to fuse and keep clear by exercising positive or negative vergence independent of accommodation. One type of stereoscope uses mirrors mounted on an adjustable mid-line barrier to control what each eye sees when both eyes are open (Figure 8.2). This is called a *Variable-Mirror*, or *Wheatstone, Stereoscope.* The other uses lenses and a nonmovable barrier between the two eyes to accomplish the same end (Figure 8.3). This is known as a *Brewster stereoscope,* also called a Biopter by one manufacturer. As such, the former allows for the separation between targets to be changed by altering the location of the mirrors; the latter requires that different target separations be presented for different prismatic demands—much like the aperture rule, above.

There is another, less obvious difference between the two: The mirror stereoscope presents near targets only; far-point fixation can be simulated only by having the patient look through plus lenses that relax accommodation. The Brewster stereoscope is more versatile in this respect. It has the capacity to simulate both near and distance viewing conditions without employing auxiliary spherical lenses. This special feature may be very useful with certain patients.

The Variable-Mirror Stereoscope is accompanied by a variety of targets. Some require first-degree fusion only; that is, they present a different, nonconflicting stimulus to each eye—the fish and bowl, for example, or the bird and cage. Some require second-degree fusion; that is, the stimulus presented to each eye is different, one from the other, but they have some features in common. Finally, there are the third-degree fusion targets. These pairs are very similar in appearance, but certain details in them are positioned so that when the overall targets are fused, the right and left eye images are not completely in register. These disparate details within the binocularly fused field produces the illusion of depth—stereopsis; for example, the targets containing eccentric rectangles or circles.

The separation of the targets is controlled by the positioning of the stereoscope's mirror panels. The manufacturer supplies a ruler that measures the prismatic demand produced by the separation of the panels. Hence, if the ruler shows the panels to be at the ortho position, it indicates that for all practical purposes the patient—if he has orthophoria at near point—will fuse the targets without exercising any positive or negative relative convergence. When the separation of the mirror panels is increased, a base-in demand is created: fusion requires an increase in negative relative convergence. When the separation of the mirror panels is reduced, the opposite effect is created. As such, because positive relative convergence typically causes the patient to feel as though he is working harder, and negative relative convergence generally requires an attitude of relaxation, it may be useful to have the patient assume a lean-over-the-task posture when working on increasing base-out ranges, and a sit-

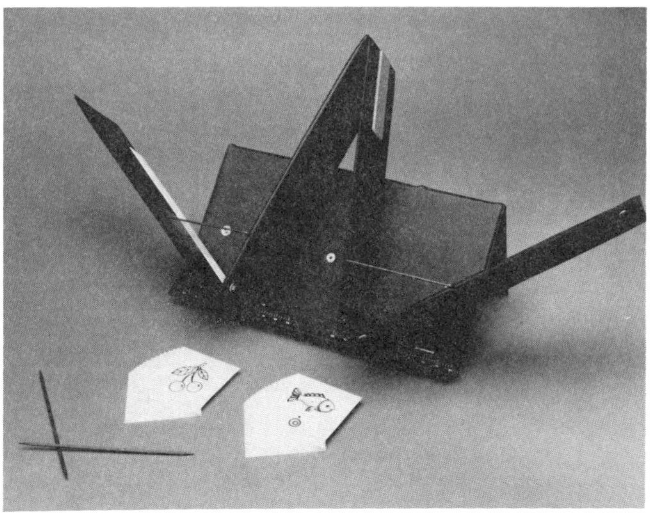

FIGURE 8.2 Variable-Mirror, or Wheatstone, Stereoscope

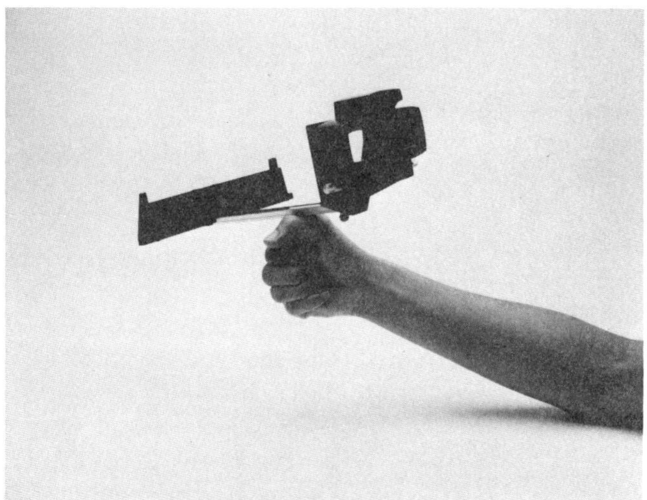

FIGURE 8.3 Brewster Stereoscope

back-and-relax posture when attempting to increase base-in abilities. (Obviously, plus and minus spherical lenses may also be introduced, thereby requiring the patient to exercise or inhibit accommodation at the same time he is learning how to increase vergence ranges.)

There are many different sets of targets available for the Brewster stereoscope. The ones called for by the procedures contained in this volume are all designed to simulate far-point fixation conditions, and all call for third-degree fusion. Three are designed to provide a base-out demand (procedures 5, 6, and 12); the other two, a base-in demand (procedures 7 and 13). All of these start off with the targets positioned so that no positive or negative relative convergence is required to fuse the two targets if the patient is orthophoric at distance. This is accomplished by having an 85 mm center-to-center separation between the pair of targets. To increase base-out demand, the separation between targets is reduced; to increase the base-in demand, the separation is increased. In both instances, accommodation is held constant and inactive (at least in theory), because the targets are positioned at the far-point setting.

The Brewster stereoscope procedures may be modified a bit by having the patient bring the slide carrier closer to his eyes. As he does this, he introduces changes in the demands made on convergence and accommodation. Obviously, by bringing the slide carrier closer, accommodation effort is needed in order to maintain clarity. Simultaneously, there is an increase in base-in demand, produced by the fact that the fixed separation between targets is relatively increased as a function of the shorter viewing distance. Hence, bringing the slide carrier closer (sometimes called *tromboning*) creates a condition wherein the patient must activate accommodation while inhibiting convergence—a difficult condition, but sometimes worth using.

Vectograms. There are a number of different devices that fall into this category. They are all similar in that they are based on the use of polarizing material for the targets and the filters worn by the patient, thereby making it possible to control what each eye sees even when both are open. This, in turn, makes it possible to stimulate positive or negative relative convergence by altering the disparity—the extent to which the targets are out of register—while keeping accommodation constant or, if spherical lenses are used, while placing a different demand on accommodation. They differ in that some use *fixed-disparity targets*, others, *variable-disparity*. In other words, some—the variable-disparity types—are made of two separate polarized plates that may be placed into relationship with each other so as to create a crossed-disparity condition (base-out demand) or an uncrossed-disparity condition (base-in demand) of a varying but controlled amount (e.g., minivectograms; see Figure 8.4). The fixed-disparity types, in contrast, are just that—fixed—with the type and amount of disparity predetermined by the manufacturer's specifications (e.g., the TV Trainer).

Tranaglyphs. These are identical, in principle, to the vectographic devices except for the fact that color takes the place of polarization as the method for controlling what is seen by each eye when both eyes are open. One target is green; the other, red; and the patient wears a red filter in front of one eye and a green filter in front of the other. (Both targets may also contain some black lines. If they do, these will be seen by both eyes. The red-green filters will not mask them.) Included in this category are the variable and nonvariable tranaglyphs such as the red/green stereo trainer, TV Trainer, minitranaglyph, etc.

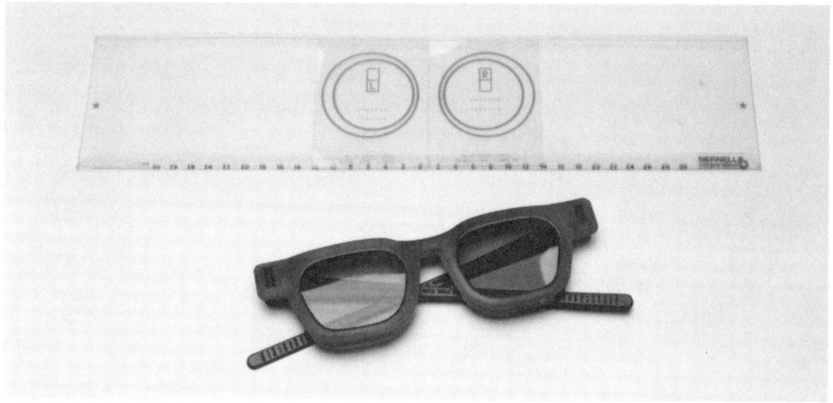

FIGURE 8.4 Horizontal Minivectograms Kit

TV Trainer. This device (Figure 8.5) employs *anaglyphic* (red-green) filters. (There is also one manufactured that employs polarizing material; it functions identically to the one described here.) It comprises a single plastic sheet, part of which is all red, another portion, all green. These are surrounded by clear plastic on which appear red and green letters and sets of red and green eccentric rings. The plastic sheet is attached to a TV screen by means of a suction cup. (It could also be placed over a window, a mirror, a newspaper, etc., if desired.) The patient wears compatible red-green filters that control what each eye sees, even though both eyes are open. The patient with single, simultaneous, binocular vision will see through the red and green sections at the same time; none of the TV screen will be blacked-out. He will also see all of the red and green letters and will perceive the illusion of depth produced by the eccentric rings. The patient who is able to obtain normal binocular vision from a certain distance (i.e., near, far) from the TV screen will be able to start his activity at that location and strive to extend his fusional ranges by moving closer or farther away from the screen. In addition, the patient may be supplied with spherical or prismatic lenses that will alter the demand on vergence and accommodation. As such, the TV Trainer is a versatile device that does not require a great deal of instruction in order to use; this makes it particularly useful with young children.

Red-Green Stereo Trainer. This device (Figure 8.6) resembles the TV Trainer except that instead of presenting solid red and green fields, its central target is an anaglyphic circle within an uncolored circle. As a result, it provides the patient who has sufficient stereopsis with an illusion of depth, with the smaller (anaglyphic) circle appearing to be in front of or behind the larger (uncolored) circle, depending upon which eye is looking through the red and which through the green filter. The red-green stereo trainer, like the TV Trainer, is versatile in that the patient can easily move from a distant to a near viewing distance.

Cheiroscope. There are three types of cheiroscopes available. All share the same main characteristic. They make it possible to present a stimulus to one eye and provide a drawing table before the partner eye where the binocular patient may project and trace over that stimulus. This makes the cheiroscope a useful device in the treatment of unilateral amblyopia manifesting in a binocular patient.

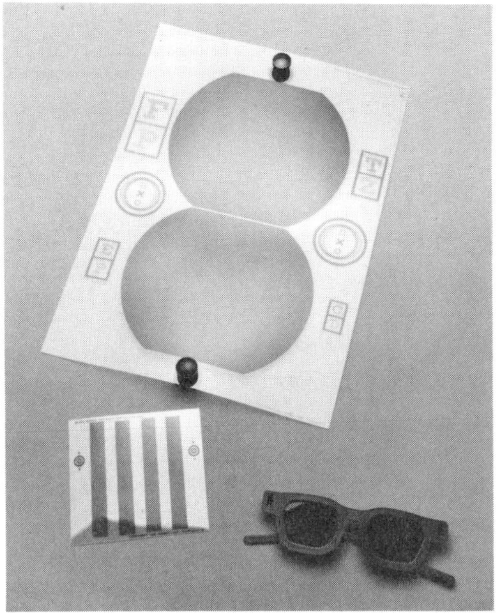

FIGURE 8.5 T.V. Trainer

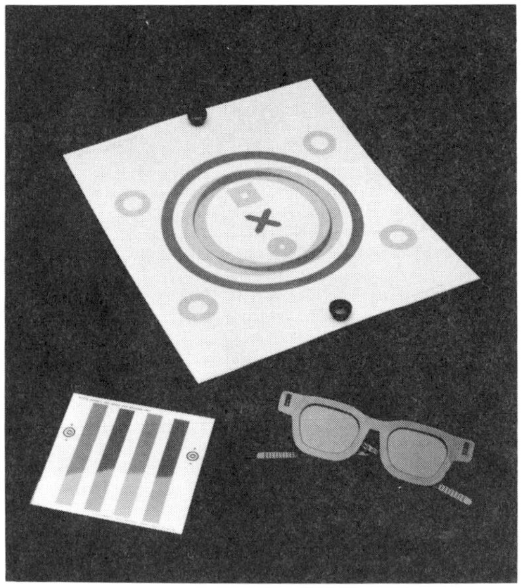

FIGURE 8.6 900 Series Red-Green Stereo Trainer

1. *Variable-Mirror Stereoscope* This device, already described above, may be converted into a cheiroscope by changing its configuration in accord with the manufacturer's easy-to-follow directions. When the device is assembled properly, the patient will be able to look into one of the stereoscope mirrors with one eye, look down on a sheet of blank paper with the other eye—the eye that is on the same side as the patient's preferred (drawing) hand—and see projected on that paper a line drawing that, in fact, is visible only to the eye looking into the mirror. He is then given a colored pencil (to make his lines more visible in contrast with the black lines of the drawing) and asked to trace over the picture. As he does this, he will be stimulating one eye under binocular viewing conditions.

2. *Single-Mirror Stereoscope* This device functions more or less like the Variable-Mirror Stereoscope. It simply looks different and is not so versatile as the latter. A visual stimulus is presented to one eye, a blank sheet of paper is placed before the partner eye (the eye that is on the same side as the patient's preferred hand), and the patient is asked to trace over the stimulus that he perceives on the paper (see Figure 8.7).

3. *Brewster Stereoscope/Cheiroscope* This device employs the same stereoscope described above but replaces the slide carrier with a drawing board. A visual stimulus is placed before one of the patient's eyes, a blank sheet of paper before the other eye—again, the eye that is on the same side as the patient's drawing hand—and the patient is asked to trace the picture.

Eccentric Rectangles. These are not actually instruments; they are merely two cards—targets—each of which has printed on it a pair of rectangles, the smaller (inner) one being located off center. The larger ones are for far-point activities; the smaller ones for near. The patient is taught how to exercise positive and negative relative convergence without an instrument, using the eccentric rectangles as targets

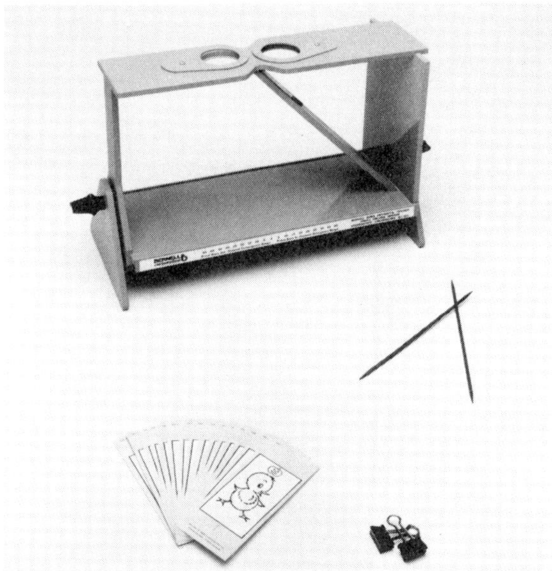

FIGURE 8.7 Single-Mirror Stereoscope

(see Figures 8.8 and 8.9). It is a demanding activity because he has to ignore the extra images that are generated under such conditions. With the standard aperture rule, the aperture slides mask these extra images from the patient's view; with the stereoscope, it is the barrier (septum) between the two eyes that accomplishes this; with the tranaglyph and vectographic devices, it is the filters that control what each eye sees. Thus, the eccentric rectangles procedures (3-I, II, III) require greater sophistication and concentration from the patient. For this reason, they are typically introduced after the patient has mastered the same kind of activity with an instrument.

It is possible for you to produce your own near and distance targets.

1. *Paper.* This is very simple to do. Simply copy pages 108 and 109 in the procedures manual, then cut these apart (into pairs) for distribution to patients. These pages may also be reproduced by an offset printer; this will cost a bit more, perhaps, but yield a more professional-looking product.

2. *Transparent.* These, too, may be made by copying pages 108 and 109. (The former are for near-point use; the latter for far-point.) Instead of photocopying the patterns onto paper, reproduce them on transparency material; then cut these apart into pairs. They are especially useful for those patients who have difficulty mastering the near-point orthopic fusion procedure and for all patients when engaged in the far-point procedures (procedure 3-II and 3-III).

3. *Tranaglyph.* Obtain a green pencil (e.g., Eagle Prismacolor Green Bice 913) and a red pencil (e.g., Eagle Prismacolor Scarlet Red 922) from an office supply or art supply dealer. Also, obtain sheets of buff-colored construction paper (i.e., the color of a standard manila mailing envelope) and a template for drawing the two sizes of rectangles. With these, the office assistant can produce anaglyphic eccentric targets that will be compatible with the anaglyphic filters listed in Table 8.1.

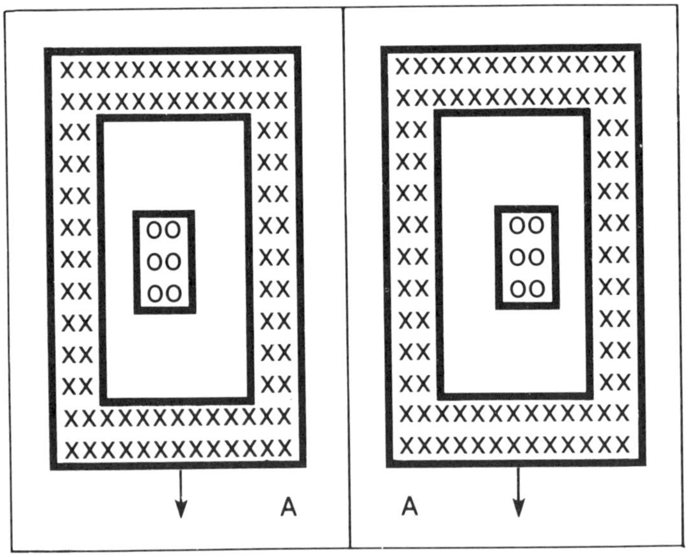

FIGURE 8.8 Near-Point Eccentric Rectangle Targets

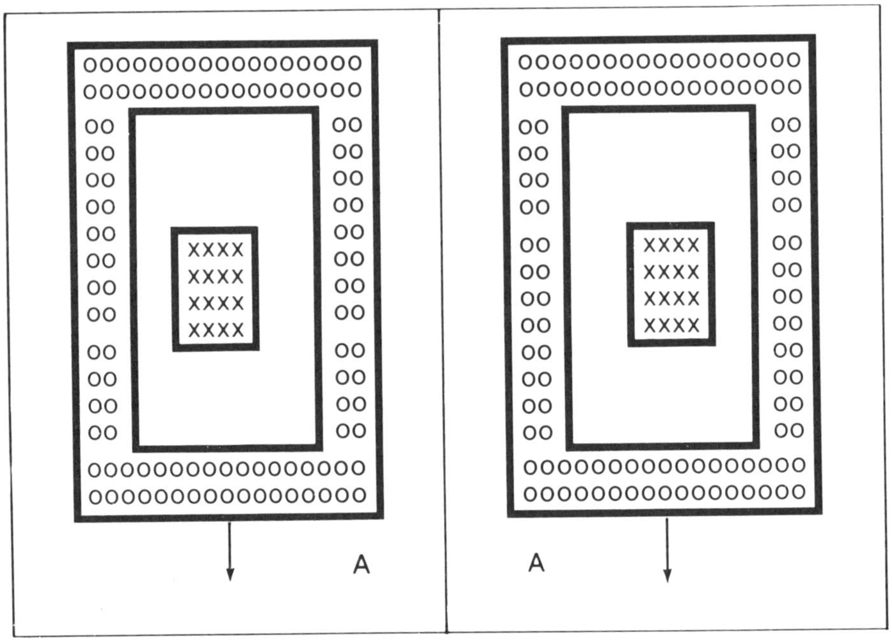

FIGURE 8.9 Far-Point Eccentric Rectangle Targets

It is also feasible to use targets other than eccentric rectangles. For example, old stereoscope cards work very well. Simply cut them in half, thereby producing a pair of stimuli in which the overall fields are identical but some of the internal details are disparate. Hence, when fused (by exercising chiastopic or orthopic fusion), the patient obtains a central, fused image that has the illusion of depth. (As a matter of fact, the illusion of depth is not really necessary. Any matched pair of targets will work, including the patient's own right and left thumbs. The drawback in not having the illusion of depth: the patient who has not yet achieved the level in his therapy where he knows when he is fusing the targets correctly will not have quite the degree of feedback he might need to monitor his own performance accurately.)

Phy-Dip Stick. This simple instrument consists of a thin metal rod, 20 in long, that is attached to a plastic handle. Mounted on the rod are three movable colored beads. This device is useful in sensitizing the patient to physiological diplopia (see procedure 21).

Lens Holder. This device serves the same purpose as the flipper frame but with more versatility. In effect, it comprises two or more lens cells on a single handle. The cells accept trial lenses, which may be easily inserted and removed.

Equipment Management

There are several ways to distribute equipment to patients. Essentially, the decision to be made is whether to sell, rent, lend, or simply give the equipment away. Rarely is a device used by a patient for more than a month; hence, purchase is not very desirable. Rental is feasible, but it has a commercial flavor that we do not find appealing. In our judgment, a combination of lending and giving away is the most satisfactory: lending when the equipment does not touch the face or is made of material that can be thoroughly cleaned before passing it on to another patient (e.g., stereoscope, vectograms); giving away when these conditions are not present (filter glasses, etc.). Such a method involves costs, of course. Even the devices that are lent will deteriorate over time and have to be replaced. The solution is to incorporate replacement costs into the office fee structure so that equipment replacement can be done without imposing a significant burden on the office budget.

Lending. The lending process works with minimum effort if the following sequence is followed:

1. When an instrument is dispensed to a patient, he should be advised that there is no charge for its use so long as it is returned in more or less the same condition as it is on the day it is lent to him. He should also be told that if it is damaged through misuse, there will be a charge; specifically, the cost of the device itself (advise the patient of this amount).
2. Enter a charge in the patient's account for the full cost of the device, but inform the patient that, should they receive a statement for services before they are scheduled to return the device, they are to ignore that charge.

3. Credit the patient's account for the full cost of the device when it is returned if it is in more or less the same condition as it was when it was given to him. If it has been damaged to the point that it needs to be replaced, leave the charge on the account and inform the patient that he is now liable for that amount. Take an instrument out of circulation when it begins to show signs of wear. No one likes to handle worn devices, particularly when they are held so close to the face.

4. This method allows one to keep track of equipment with minimum effort. If an open account (one showing a balance due) shows an equipment charge, and the date of that charge is past the time when the device should have been returned, simply bill it and consider it sold.

FEES

Fees will vary from region to region, let alone from office to office within the same region. But, regardless of this variance, fees should reflect professional time and effort.

There are certain options to be considered when establishing fees. Some optometrists prefer to set a fee on the basis of the condition that is being treated; in a way, similar to the orthodontist. Hence, the fee remains fixed, even though the time required to treat the condition successfully may vary somewhat. Others prefer to establish fees on a per-visit basis. A third option is a merging of the two: a certain set amount that reflects the nature of the condition to be treated; this accompanied by a per-visit fee that reflects the time required to accomplish the goal. In our opinion, the second—per-visit—basis is most desirable for both the patient and the practitioner, especially in this era when third-party payments are becoming more common.

EFFECTIVE USE OF OFFICE SPACE

Incorporating vision therapy into a primary-care practice does not require the allocation of very much extra space. Most offices already have space outside of the examination room(s) devoted to such instruments as perimeter, tonometer, tangent screen, and automated refractor, and such services as teaching patients how to manage their contact lenses. There is no reason why the vision therapy program cannot be conducted within one of these same areas. All that is needed, in most cases, is sufficient space to accommodate the office assistant, a patient, and a parent. (It is desirable, although not essential, to have a window in this area so that the patient has the option to direct his gaze to infinity while carrying out orthopic fusion procedures.) It is also convenient to have office-based, demonstration instruments situated in a permanent location so that the patient can be shown what to do at home without having to handle the device he will be taking home, but it is not necessary. Instruments and materials may be housed in a conveniently located closet and assembled as needed. For that matter, this latter option may be preferable, inasmuch as the patient will have to know how to assemble the instrument when he prepares to engage in the procedures at home.

Bibliography

BINOCULAR ANOMALIES

Burian H, von Noorden G. *Binocular vision and ocular motility.* (3d ed). St. Louis: CV Mosby, 1985.

Griffin J. *Binocular anomalies: Procedures for vision therapy.* New York: Professional Press Books, 1982.

Parks MM. *Ocular motility and strabismus.* New York: Harper & Row, 1975.

Pickwell D. *Binocular vision anomalies: Investigation and treatment.* Boston: Butterworths, 1984.

Rosner J. *Pediatric optometry.* Boston: Butterworths, 1982.

CHILD DEVELOPMENT

Frankenburg WK, Goldstein AD, Camp BW. The revised Denver Developmental Screening Test: Its accuracy as a screening test. *Journal Pediatr* 1971; 79(6):988–995.

Gesell A, Halverson HM, Thompson H, Igl FL, Castner BM, Ames LB, Armatruda CS. *The first five years of life: A guide to the study of the preschool child.* New York: Harper & Row, 1940.

Ilg FL, Ames LB. *School readiness.* New York: Harper & Row, 1965.

LEARNING DISABILITIES AND DYSLEXIA

Duffy FH, Geschwind N (eds). *Dyslexia: A neuroscientific approach to clinical evaluation.* Boston: Little, Brown & Co., 1985.

Levine MD, Brooks R, Shonkoff JP (eds). *A pediatric approach to learning disorders.* New York: John Wiley & Sons, 1980.

Mauser AJ. *Assessing the learning disabled.* Novato, Calif.: Academic Therapy Publications, 1981.

Miles TR. *Dyslexia, the pattern of difficulties.* New York: Granada, 1983.

Money J, Schiffman G (eds). *The disabled reader: Education of the dyslexic child.* Baltimore: Johns Hopkins Press, 1966.

Pavlides GT, Miles TR. *Dyslexia research and its application to education.* New York: John Wiley and Sons, 1981.

Solan H (ed). *The treatment and management of children with learning disabilities.* Springfield, Ill: CS Thomas, 1982.

PERCEPTUAL SKILLS AND SCHOOL PERFORMANCE

Bender L. *A visual motor gestalt test and its clinical uses.* New York: Am.Orthopsych.Assn., 1938.

Bradley L, Bryant PE. Categorizing sounds and learning to read: A causal connection. *Nature* 1983;301,419–421.

Bryant P. *Perception and understanding in young children: An experimental approach*. New York: Basic Books, 1974.

Carter DB. Vision and learning disorders. In Carter DB (ed). *Approaches to learning disorders*. Philadelphia: Chilton Books, 1970.

Dong D. Relationships among copy form tests. Unpublished thesis. School of Optometry, University of California Berkeley, 1978.

Foorman, BR, Non-alphabetic codes in learning to read: The case of the Japanese. In Foorman, BR, Siegel AW (eds). *Acquisition of reading skills: Cultural constraints and cognitive universals*. Hillsdale, NJ: Lawrence Erlbaum Associates, 1986.

Gagne R. *The conditions of learning*. 2d ed. New York: Holt, Rinehart & Winston, 1970.

Hein A, Jeannerod M (eds). *Spatially oriented behavior*. New York: Springer-Verlag, 1983.

Helveston E, Ellis FD, Weber JC, Helveston BH, Miller K. Performance test to accompany ophthalmic examination in the young school age child: The "draw a bicycle" test. *J Pediatr Ophthalmol Strab* 1985;22:17–19.

Klein, SD. *Psychological testing of children*. Boston: Exceptional Parent Press, 1977.

Lewkowicz N. Phonemic awareness training: What to teach and how to teach it. *J Ed Psyc* 1980;72:686–700.

Liberman IY, Shankweiler D, Liberman AM, Fowler C, Fischer FW. Phonetic segmentation and recoding in the beginning reader. In Reber AS, Scarborough DL (eds). *Toward a psychology of reading*. Hillsdale, N.J.: Lawrence Erlbaum Associates, 1980.

McInnis P. *McInnis/Hammondsport Plan*. New York: Walker Educational Book Corp, 1977.

Rosner J. *Helping children overcome learning difficulties*. 2d ed. New York: Walker Publishing Co, 1979.

Rosner J. Individualization of instruction. In Connors FP, et al. (eds). *Professional preparation of educators of crippled children*. New York: Teachers College Press, 1970.

Rosner J. Screening for perceptual skills dysfunction: An update. *JAOA* 1979;50(10):1115–1119.

Rosner J. Language arts and arithmetic achievement, and specifically related perceptual skills. *Am Ed Res J* 1973;10(1):59–68.

Rosner J. Perceptual development. In Gottlieb J, Strichart SS (eds). *Developmental theory and research in learning disabilities*. Baltimore: University Park Press, 1981.

Rosner J. Phonological skills and learning to read and write: Reactions and implications. In Foorman B, Siegel A (eds). *Acquisition of reading skills: Cultural constraints and cognitive universals*. Hillsdale, NJ: Lawrence Erlbaum Associates, 1986.

Rosner J. Visual analysis training and the copying skills of four-year-old children. Learning Research and Development Center, University of Pittsburgh.

Rosner J. Individual differences in perceptual skills: Identification, modification and effects. *Proceedings of the American Psychological Assn 80th meeting*.

Rosner J. Auditory analysis training with pre-readers. *The Reading Teacher* 1974;27(4):379–384.

Rosner J. Visual analysis training with preschool children. *JAOA* 1974;45(5):584–591.

Rosner J, Gruber J. Differences in the perceptual skills development of young myopes and hyperopes. *Am J Optom Physiol Opt* 1985;62:501–504.

Rosner J, Rosner J. Management of perceptual skills disorders in a primary care practice. *JAOA* 1986;57:56–59.

Rosner J, Simon D. The auditory analysis test: An initial report. *Journal of Learning Disabilities* 1971;4(7):384–392.

Solan HA, Groffman S. Understanding and treating developmental and perceptual motor disabilities. In Solan HA (ed). *The treatment and management of children with learning disabilities*. Springfield, Ill: CS Thomas, 1982.

Weaver P, Rosner J. Relationships between visual and auditory perceptual skill and comprehension independent of decoding. *J Learning Disabilities* 1979;12(9):617–621.

TESTS

Bender Visual-Motor Gestalt Test for Children
Western Psychological Services
P.O. Box 775
Beverly Hills, CA 90213

Denver Developmental Screening Test
DDM
P.O. Box 20037
Denver, CO 80220

Developmental Test of Visual-Motor Integration
Follett Educational Corp.
P.O. Box 5705
Chicago, IL 60680

Lindamood Auditory Conceptualization Test
Teaching Resources Corp.
50 Pond Park Rd.
Hingham, MA 02043

Rutgers Drawing Test
A. Starr
126 Montgomery St.
Highland Park, NJ 08904

Slosson Drawing Coordination Test
Slosson Educational Publications
140 Pine St.
East Aurora, NY 14052

Wepman Auditory Discrimination Test (revised)
Language Research Associates
950 E. 59th St.
Chicago, IL 60621

Winter Haven Kindergarten Perceptual Testing Kit
Special Educational Materials, Inc.
484 S. Broadway
Yonkers, NY 10705

PERCEPTUAL SKILLS TRAINING PROGRAMS

DLM Teaching Resources
P.O. Box 4000
Allen, TX 75002

Educators Publishing Service
75 Moulton St.
Cambridge, MA 02138

Walker Educational Book Corp.
727 Fifth Avenue
New York, NY 10019

COMPENSATORY INSTRUCTION

Glaser R, Rosner J. Toward the design of adaptive environments for learning. In Talmadge H (ed). *Individualized instruction systems.* Chicago: National Society of Studies in Education, 1975.

Money J, Schiffman G (eds). *The disabled reader: Education of the dyslexic child.* Baltimore: Johns Hopkins Press, 1966.

Resnick L, Wang M, Rosner J. Adaptive education for young children: The Primary Education Project. In Day MC, Parker RK (eds). *The preschool in action.* 2d ed. Boston: Allyn & Bacon, 1975.

Rosner J. Teaching hard-to-teach children to read: A rationale for compensatory education. In Resnick L, Weaver P (eds). *Reading theories and practices.* Hillsdale, NJ: Lawrence Erlbaum Associates, 1977.

Rosner J. The use of tests in an adaptive instructional environment. In Wilson A (ed). *Assessment for the teaching/learning process.* Toronto: Ontario Institute for Studies in Education, 1984.

Treiman R, Baron J. Phonemic-analysis training helps children benefit from spelling-sound rules. *Memory & Cognition* 1983;11:382–389.

Williams J. Teaching decoding with an emphasis on phoneme analysis and phoneme blending. *J Ed Psych* 1980;71:1–15.

Index